KIDNEY DISEASE

RECIPES

COOKBOOK

Delicious and Healthful Recipes for Kidney Wellness

FRED G. MORRIS

Copyright © 2023 FRED G. MORRIS

TABLE OF CONTENTS

UNDERSTANDING KIDNEY DISEASE

Renal disease, commonly referred to as kidney disease, is a disorder when the kidneys do not work correctly. The kidneys are important organs that are in charge of eliminating extra fluid from the body and filtering waste from the blood. Waste products accumulate in the body when the kidneys are not working correctly, which may lead to some health issues.

Numerous variables, including genetics, illnesses, and way of life choices, might contribute to kidney disease. It is a severe medical disorder that over time may cause kidney function to decline. They produce hormones that promote the development of red blood cells.

The inability of the kidneys to function correctly as a result of injury or illness may result in a variety of symptoms and problems. The body's filtration and elimination systems depend heavily on the kidneys, a pair of organs situated in the abdominal cavity.

They are in charge of eliminating extra salt, water, and waste from the blood as well as preserving the body's electrolyte and other chemical balances. However, renal disease may impair kidney function, resulting in toxin accumulation, fluid overload, and electrolyte abnormalities in the body. To stop additional damage and properly treat renal disease, early detection is crucial.

TYPES OF KIDNEY DISEASES

✓ *Acute Kidney Injury (AKI)*

Acute Kidney Injury (AKI) is the term used to describe a quick and fast reduction in kidney function that is often brought on by kidney damage or injury. With timely medical care, this form of kidney illness may often be treated.

✓ *Chronic Kidney Disease (CKD)*

Over time, the kidneys lose their capacity to operate normally as a result of chronic kidney disease (CKD). Other medical disorders including high blood pressure, diabetes, or heart disease are often the root cause of CKD. CKD may develop into end-stage renal disease (ESRD) if it is not addressed.

✓ *Renal end-stage disease (ESRD)*

The last stage of kidney illness, known as end-stage renal disease (ESRD), occurs when the kidneys are entirely incapable of functioning. Dialysis or a kidney transplant is necessary for ESRD patients to live.

KIDNEY DISEASE CAUSES

✓ *Diabetes*

Diabetes is a disease in which the body struggles to control blood sugar levels. Kidney illness may result from high blood sugar levels harming the blood arteries in the kidneys.

✓ *Elevated Blood Pressure*

Kidney disease may be brought on by high blood pressure, often known as hypertension, which damages the blood vessels in the kidneys.

✓ *Genetic Influences*

Genetic factors may contribute to some kidney diseases, such as polycystic kidney disease.

✓ *Autoimmune Conditions*

Renal inflammation brought on by autoimmune conditions like lupus may result in renal damage.

✓ *Infections*

Infections may harm the kidneys and result in kidney disease, such as glomerulonephritis.

Acute Kidney Disease Symptoms

Depending on the underlying cause and the stage of the illness, the symptoms of kidney disease might change. Kidney illness is sometimes referred to be a "silent" disease since in its early stages, it may not show any symptoms at all. But when the condition worsens, symptoms might start to appear.

Acute kidney disease symptoms may range from the following and can appear over a few hours to days:

✓ Reduced urine production: One of the most typical signs of acute renal illness is a reduction in urine production. The body's ability to generate urine may be impaired or nonexistent. This is because the kidneys are in charge of filtering waste from the blood and generating urine.

✓ Swelling, commonly referred to as edema, is another typical sign of acute renal illness. Legs, feet, ankles, or the face may all swell up. This is because the kidneys are in charge of controlling the body's fluid balance. Swelling may result from an accumulation of extra fluid in the body when the kidneys are not working correctly.

✓ Fatigue, often known as excessive weariness or exhaustion, is a common symptom of acute renal illness. This is because erythropoietin, a hormone produced by the kidneys that promotes the creation of red blood cells, is what causes the kidneys to produce red blood cells. Anemia and weariness may result from the body not producing enough erythropoietin when the kidneys are not working correctly.

✓ Vomiting and nausea: Acute renal illness might also induce these symptoms. This is because the kidneys are in charges of filtering waste materials from the blood, such as poisons and extra fluid. These waste products may accumulate in the body and cause nausea and vomiting when the kidneys are not working correctly.

✓ Breathlessness: Breathlessness is another sign of acute renal illness. This is because the kidneys are in charge of eliminating extra fluid from the body. It may be challenging to breathe when the kidneys are not working correctly because extra fluid can build up in the lungs.

✓ Confusion: Disorientation or confusion are additional symptoms of acute renal illness. This is because the kidneys are in charge of clearing toxins from the blood. These poisons may accumulate in the body when the kidneys are not working correctly, which can cause confusion or disorientation.

✓ Chest discomfort: Acute renal illness may sometimes induce chest pain. This is because the kidneys are in charge of controlling the body's electrolyte balance, which includes potassium levels. Potassium levels may become too high when the kidneys are not working correctly, which can cause chest discomfort or heart palpitations.

✓ Hypertension: Acute renal illness may also result in elevated blood pressure, generally known as hypertension. This is because the kidneys, which are in charge of manufacturing hormones that regulate blood vessel constriction and dilatation, are also in charge of controlling blood pressure. Blood pressure may rise when the kidneys are not working correctly.

The following are possible kidney disease treatments

✓ ***Medication:*** Drugs may be administered to treat kidney disease symptoms including high blood pressure, anemia, and excessive potassium levels in the blood. To halt the spread of the condition, medication may sometimes be recommended.

✓ ***Changes in food and lifestyle:*** Eating healthily and keeping a healthy weight may help control the signs and symptoms of renal disease. Patients could be instructed to consume fewer items, such as salt and protein while consuming more fruits and vegetables. Reduced alcohol consumption and giving up smoking may also be advised.

✓ ***Dialysis:*** Dialysis is a medical procedure in which waste materials are removed from the blood using a machine. Hemodialysis, which is carried out in a hospital or dialysis facility, and peritoneal dialysis, which is carried out at home, are the two forms of dialysis. Patients with ESRD may be advised to undergo dialysis.

✓ Transplanting a patient's damaged kidney with a healthy kidney from a donor is known as a kidney transplant. Patients with ESRD who are otherwise healthy enough to have the surgery are often the only ones who can get a kidney transplant.

✓ Patients with kidney illness may benefit from working with a team of healthcare experts, such as a nutritionist, a social worker, and a nephrologist (a specialist in kidney disorders), in addition to receiving medical therapy. These experts can provide encouragement and direction throughout therapy and assist patients in coping with the mental and physical difficulties associated with having renal disease.

KIDNEY DISEASE AND DIET

The Impact of Diet on Kidney Disease

For controlling renal illness and maintaining kidney function, a good diet is essential. The stress on the kidneys may be lessened and additional damage can be avoided with the appropriate diet. The following are some ways that nutrition might impact renal disease:

✓ ***Salt:*** A diet heavy in salt may raise blood pressure, which harms the kidneys. Aim for a daily salt consumption of fewer than 2,300 milligrams for those with renal disease.

✓ ***Protein:*** Protein is necessary for the body's tissue growth and repair, but too much protein may damage the kidneys. Protein breakdown results in waste products that the kidneys must filter out of the body. Protein consumption for those with renal disease should be kept to 0.8 grams per kilogram of body weight per day.

✓ Potassium is a mineral that aids in controlling the body's fluid balance. For those with renal illness, however, too much potassium might be hazardous since the kidneys might not be able to eliminate too much potassium from the blood. Those who have renal illness should try to keep their daily potassium consumption between 2,000 and 3,000 milligrams.

✓ For strong bones and teeth, phosphorus is a necessary mineral. For those with renal illness, however, too much phosphorus might be dangerous since the kidneys might not be able to eliminate too much phosphorus from the blood. For those who have renal disease, the recommended daily phosphorus intake ranges from 800 to 1,000 milligrams.

✓ *Fluids:* People with renal illness may have negative effects from having too much fluid in their bodies because their kidneys may not be able to clear the extra fluid from the body. Fluid consumption for those with renal illness should be kept at 1.5 to 2 liters per day.

<u>*The Best Diet For Those With Kidney Disease Is*</u>

The optimal diet for those with renal disease should be low in fluids, salt, protein, potassium, and phosphorus. Dietary therapies are one of the most efficient strategies to manage CKD since they may lessen symptoms, halt the disease's development, and enhance general health outcomes.

✓ *Reduce Your Protein Intake*

A high-protein diet may put more strain on the kidneys, which might make CKD worse. As a result, it is recommended that people with renal illness cut down on their protein consumption. A protein intake of 0.6–0.8 grams per kilogram of body weight per day is advised for those with CKD. Processed meats and fast meals should be avoided in favor of high-quality protein sources such as lean meats, fish, eggs, and dairy products.

✓ *Limit your sodium intake.*

Consuming too much salt may raise blood pressure, which worsens kidney disease. Therefore, it is suggested that those who have CKD limit their salt consumption.

Less than 2,300 milligrams of salt per day is the recommended daily consumption. Fresh fruits and vegetables should be eaten instead of items rich in salt such as canned goods, processed meals, and fast food.

✓ *Watch your intake of phosphorus and potassium.*

An accumulation of potassium and phosphorus in the blood may occur in people with CKD, which may lead to significant consequences. It is crucial to monitor and restrict the consumption of these minerals.

Potassium should be consumed in amounts of 2,000 to 2,500 milligrams per day, while phosphorus should be consumed in amounts of 800 to 1,000 milligrams per day. Bananas, avocados, tomatoes, almonds, and dairy products are examples of foods rich in potassium and phosphorus that should be taken in moderation.

✓ *Increase Fruit and Vegetable Intake*

The vitamins, minerals, and antioxidants found in fruits and vegetables are crucial for the kidneys' health. It is recommended that people with CKD eat 3-5 servings of fruits and vegetables daily. However, certain fruits and vegetables, including tomatoes, oranges, potatoes, and spinach, are rich in potassium and should be eaten in moderation.

✓ *Pick healthy fats.*

Monounsaturated and polyunsaturated fats are examples of good fats that may help decrease inflammation and enhance overall health.

For those with CKD, the omega-3 fatty acids in fish, nuts, and seeds are very advantageous. However, processed meals, fried foods, and fast food should all be avoided since they include saturated and trans fats.

✓ *Consume A Lot of Water*

Water consumption may aid in the body's removal of waste materials and toxins, which can enhance kidney function. It is recommended that people with CKD consume 8 to 10 glasses of water daily. But those who have severe renal illness may need to restrict their fluid consumption.

✓ *Don't drink or use tobacco.*

Smoking and drinking may raise blood pressure and further harm the kidneys. As a result, those who have CKD are recommended to abstain from or reduce their cigarette and alcohol use.

CHAPTER 1

RECIPES FOR BREAKFAST AND BRUNCH

SCRAMBLED VEGETABLE AND EGG

There are 2 servings in this recipe.

Cooking time: This meal takes between 10 and 15 minutes to prepare.

Preparation: This dish requires around 5 to 10 minutes of preparation.

About 190 calories, 13 grams of protein, 12 grams of fat, and 6 grams of carbs are included in each meal.

- *4 eggs*
- *14 cups finely chopped onion, 14 cups finely chopped bell pepper, and 14 cup finely chopped mushrooms*
- *Olive oil, 1 tbsp.*
- *Pepper and salt as desired*

Makings:

- *The eggs should be beaten with a fork in a basin before being placed aside.*

- *In a nonstick skillet over medium heat, warm the olive oil.*
- *When the veggies are ready, add the chopped onion, bell pepper, and mushrooms to the pan and cook for 3–4 minutes.*

- *After adding the beaten eggs, mix the veggies.*

- *Cook the eggs for a further few minutes, stirring periodically, until they are no longer runny.*

- *To taste, add salt and pepper to the food.*

- *Serving hot, please.*

Vegetable and egg scramble is a tasty and convenient breakfast item that is also nutrient-dense. You may have a nutritious and filling supper that will keep you energized for the rest of the day by following the recipe above.

OATMEAL WITH BLUEBERRIES

This dish takes 15 minutes to cook and 2 minutes to prep, and it feeds 2 people.

Dietary information (per serving)

- *260 calories*
- *Fat: 4g*
- *48g of carbohydrates*
- *6g of fiber*
- *9g protein*

Ingredients:

- *Rolled oats, 1 cup*
- *2 cups of water or milk, either dairy or vegan*
- *14 teaspoons of salt*
- *One-half teaspoon of vanilla extract*
- *1/2 cup blueberries, either fresh or frozen*
- *1 tablespoon maple syrup or honey (optional)*

<u>*Makings:*</u>

- *Combine the oats, milk or water, and salt in a medium saucepan. Over medium heat, bring to a boil while stirring periodically.*

- *When the muesli is thick and creamy, lower the heat to low and simmer for 10 to 15 minutes, stirring periodically.*

- *Add the blueberries and vanilla essence, and simmer for a further two to three minutes, or until the blueberries are heated through.*

- *Serve hot and sweeten, if preferred, with honey or maple syrup.*

- *Due to its high fiber and protein content, blueberry muesli is a substantial and fulfilling breakfast alternative.*

- *Additionally, it has a lot of antioxidants, vitamins, and minerals that support general health. You can quickly prepare a tasty and healthy breakfast by following these easy instructions.*

TOAST WITH AVOCADO AND TOMATO

Size of serving: 1

2 minutes for cooking

5 minutes to prepare

Information about diet:

- *300 calories*
- *Fat: 20g*
- *25g of carbohydrates*
- *7g protein*
- *9g of fiber*

Ingredients:

- *1 piece of bread, preferably whole grain or sourdough*
- *12 an avocado*
- *1 little tomato*
- *Pepper and salt as desired*
- *Red pepper flakes, sesame seeds, or a splash of olive oil are optional garnishes.*

Makings:

- *The bread should be crisp and gently browned after being toasted in a toaster or toaster oven.*

- *Slice the avocado in half and take out the pit while the bread is browning. Take the meat and mash it with a fork in a small basin.*

- *The tomato should be cut into thin rounds.*

- *Spread the mashed avocado evenly over the toast after it has finished toasting.*

- *On top of the avocado, arrange the tomato slices and season with salt and pepper to suit.*

- *Add whatever extras you like, such as sesame seeds or red pepper flakes, and pour some olive oil if you want.*

- *Enjoy your toast with avocado, tomato, and other nutritious ingredients.*

PARFAIT DE GREECE YOGURT

Size of serving: 1

5 minutes to prepare

0 minutes were spent cooking.

Ingredients:

- *Greek yogurt plain, half a cup*
- *Blueberries, strawberries, raspberries, and other fruit, totaling 1/2 cup*
- *Granola, 1/4 cup*
- *1 tablespoon of optional honey*

- *Greek yogurt and honey (if used) should be well blended in a small bowl.*

- *Mix the mixed berries in a separate basin.*

- *Layer the Greek yogurt mixture, mixed berries, and granola in a glass or container.*

- *Up until the glass or jar is full, keep stacking.*

- *If desired, top with more mixed berries and granola.*

- *Dispense and savor.*

Approximate Nutritional Information

- *300 calories*

- *17g of protein*

- *Fat: 6g*

- *45g of carbohydrates*

- *6g of fiber*

- *25g sugar*

Protein, fiber, and antioxidant-rich Greek yogurt parfait make a healthy and filling breakfast or snack. Additionally, it is a fantastic method to increase the amount of fruit and healthy grains in your diet. Try it, and you'll love how tasty and healthy it is!

OMELETTE WITH SPINACH AND MUSHROOMS

Portion size

One person may eat the dish.

Cooking Period

Cooking time for this dish is between 10 and 15 minutes.

Prepare Time

This dish requires around five minutes of preparation time.

Info about nutrition:

Depending on the precise ingredients and serving sizes used, this spinach and mushroom omelet has between 200 and 250 calories. Additionally, it's a fantastic source of fiber, protein, and important vitamins and minerals.

Ingredients:

- *2 eggs*
- *25% of a cup of chopped mushrooms*
- *Fresh spinach leaves, half a cup*
- *1/4 cup of cheese, shredded*
- *Pepper and salt as desired*
- *1 teaspoon olive oil*

Makings:

- *In a nonstick frying pan over medium heat, warm the olive oil.*

- *The mushrooms should be sautéed in the pan after being chopped until they are soft and slightly browned.*

- *Once the spinach leaves have wilted, add them to the pan and continue cooking.*

- *Beat the eggs with a dash of salt and pepper in another bowl.*

- *Making ensuring the eggs are spread equally, pour the beaten eggs over the mushrooms and spinach in the pan.*

- *The omelet should be cooked for 2 to 3 minutes, or until the eggs are set and the bottom is gently browned.*

- *On top of one side of the omelet, scatter the shredded cheese.*

- *The remaining half of the omelet should be carefully folded over the cheese using a spatula.*

- *Cook the omelet for a further one to two minutes, or until it is done and the cheese has melted.*

- *Enjoy your hot, tasty, and nutritious meal after serving the omelet.*

OATMEAL WITH APPLES AND CINNAMON

This recipe yields enough for two individuals.

15-20 minutes for cooking

5 minutes to prepare

<u>Dietary information (per serving):</u>

- *267 calories*
- *Fat: 5g*
- *49g of carbohydrates*
- *8g of fiber*
- *7g protein*

Ingredients:

- *Rolled oats, 1 cup*
- *2-cups of water*
- *1 cored and chopped apple*
- *12 teaspoon cinnamon*
- *14 teaspoon salt*
- *1 tablespoon (optional) maple syrup*
- *(Optional) 1/4 cup chopped nuts*

Makings:

- *Bring the water to a rolling boil in a medium saucepan.*

- *Add the salt, cinnamon, apple, and oats. To blend, stir.*

- *When the oats are cooked through and the sauce is thick and creamy, reduce the heat to medium and simmer for 10-15 minutes, stirring regularly.*

- *Add the maple syrup and chopped nuts, if preferred.*
- *Serve warm.*

Muesli with apple and cinnamon is a fantastic way to start the day with a delicious and nutritious meal. This dish is certain to become a regular in your morning rotation because of its straightforward ingredients and simple-to-follow instructions.

FRITTATA WITH TURKEY AND VEGETABLES

Servings: four

15 minutes for preparation

25 minutes for cooking

Dietary information (per serving):

- *233 calories*
- *Fat total: 11.7g*
- *3.6g of saturated fat*
- *250mg cholesterol*
- *Salt: 408 mg*
- *6.3g of total carbs*
- *1.3g of dietary fiber*
- *3.3g of sugars*
- *24.8g of protein*

Ingredients:

- ***Eight big eggs***
- ***0.5 cups of milk***
- ***1/4 tsp. of black pepper and 1/2 tsps. of salt***
- ***1 tablespoon of olive oil***
- ***One medium zucchini, one red pepper, one tiny onion, and one cup chopped cooked turkey.***
- ***1/2 cup of cheddar cheese, shredded***

Makings:

- ***Set the oven's temperature to 350°F (175°C).***

- ***Whisk the eggs, milk, salt, and pepper in a large basin.***

- ***In a large oven-safe skillet, heat the olive oil over medium heat.***

- *Add the bell pepper, zucchini, and onion. Cook for approximately 5-7 minutes, stirring periodically, or until the veggies are soft.*

- *Stir in the cooked turkey after adding it to the skillet.*

- *Gently incorporate the veggies and turkey into the egg mixture after pouring it into the pan.*

- *On top of the frittata, strew the grated cheese.*

- *When the eggs have set and the cheese is melted and golden brown, place the pan in the preheated oven and bake for 20 to 25 minutes.*

- *Before slicing and serving, remove the frittata from the oven and let it cool for a while.*

- ***To sum up, turkey and vegetable frittata is a delicious and nutritious dish that is suitable for any time of day. You can make a wonderful frittata that is loaded with veggies, protein, and flavor with this simple recipe.***

BREAKTIME BOWL OF QUINOA

Portion size

There are four servings in this recipe.

Prepare Time:

Ten minutes

Cooking Period

Two hours

- *310 calories*
- *14g of protein; 16g of fat*
- *29g of carbohydrates*
- *8g of fiber*
- *2g sugar*

Ingredients:

- *Quinoa, one cup*
- *2-cups of water*
- *4 big eggs, 1/4 teaspoon salt*
- *1 sliced avocado*
- *Half a cup of cherry tomatoes*
- *14 cups finely minced fresh cilantro*
- *Wedges sliced from 1 lime*

- *Pepper and salt as desired*

Makings:

- *Place the rinsed quinoa in a medium saucepan after straining it through a fine mesh strainer. Over high heat, add the water and salt and bring to a boil.*

- *Low heat should be used to cover the pot. For 15 to 20 minutes, or until the water is absorbed and the quinoa is cooked, simmer the quinoa.*

- *Fry the eggs in a nonstick pan over medium heat until the whites are set but the yolks are still runny while the quinoa is cooking.*

- *Allotted quinoa should be divided among four bowls. Fry an egg and place it on top of each bowl along with cherry tomatoes, avocado slices, and cilantro.*

- *Lime wedges are placed on the side of the quinoa bowls for squeezing over the top. To taste, add salt and pepper to the food.*

- *Enjoy your filling and tasty morning bowl of quinoa.*

BAGEL WITH SMOKED SALMON AND CREAM CHEESE

One serving is produced by this recipe.

No cooking is necessary for this meal, however toasting the bagel will take around 2-3 minutes.

Preparation time: This dish takes around 5-7 minutes to prepare.

<u>*Information about diet:*</u>

- *400 calories*
- *18g of protein*
- *Fat: 20g*
- *36g of carbohydrates*
- *3g of fiber*
- *Sucrose: 5g*
- *Salt: 790 mg*

<u>*Ingredients:*</u>

- *One plain bagel*
- *Smoked salmon, 2 oz.*
- *2/batch of cream cheese*
- *1 tablespoon finely minced fresh chives*

- *Pepper and salt as desired*

<u>*Makings:*</u>

- *The bagel should be lightly toasted after toasting.*

- *On both halves of the bagel, equally, distribute the cream cheese.*

- *Over the cream cheese, arrange the smoked salmon.*

- *If preferred, top with chopped chives and season with salt and pepper to taste.*

- *Your delectable bagel with cream cheese and smoked salmon is ready for serving.*

- *Advice: You may also top your bagel with thinly sliced red onion, capers, or tomato for a bit of additional flavor.*

TOAST WITH BANANAS AND ALMOND BUTTER

Portion size

There is one serving in this recipe.

This meal doesn't need any cooking time.
Preparation: This dish takes around 5 minutes to prepare.

Information about diet:

- *280 calories*

- *8g protein*

- *Fat: 12g*

- *38g of carbohydrates*

- *6g of fiber*

- *Sucrose: 13g*

- *220 mg of sodium*

Ingredients:

- *1 whole wheat piece of bread*

- *1 little banana*

- *1-tablespoon almond butter*

- *1 tsp. optional honey*

- *Cinnamon spice, optional*

Makings:

- *The bread slice should be lightly toasted after toasting.*

- *On the bread slice, evenly distribute the almond butter.*

- *Bananas should be peeled and cut into thin rounds.*

- *The almond butter is layered on top of the banana slices.*

- *If desired, drizzle honey on top of the banana slices.*

- *Adding cinnamon is optional.*

- *Toast with wonderful banana and almond butter should be served and enjoyed.*

- *Advice: You may sprinkle some chopped almonds or walnuts on top of the banana slices for more crunch. Additionally, you may want to experiment with nut butter other than almond or peanut.*

SANDWICH WITH TUNA SALAD

Size of Serving: 2 sandwiches

0 minutes were spent cooking.

10 minutes for preparation

Per-serving nutritional information:

- *340 calories*
- *Fat: 16g*
- *22g of carbohydrates*
- *28g of protein*

Ingredients:

- *1 can of drained tuna*
- *Mayonnaise, 2 tablespoons*
- *1/fourth cup of Dijon mustard*

- *Lemon juice, 1 tablespoon*

- *1 sliced celery stalk*

- *1 minced green onion*

- *Pepper and salt as desired*

- *Bread, four pieces*

- *Greens like lettuce are optional.*

Makings:

- *Tuna, mayonnaise, Dijon mustard, lemon juice, celery, and green onions should all be combined in a bowl.*

- *To taste, add salt and pepper.*

- *If desired, toast the bread pieces.*

- *On one piece of bread, arrange some lettuce or other leaves.*

- *Onto the toast, spoon the tuna salad mixture.*

- *Add the second piece of bread on top.*

- *Serve the sandwich by cutting it in half.*

- *Enjoy your tasty sandwich with tuna salad.*

DESSERT BURRITO

This recipe yields one tortilla as the serving size.

15 to 20 minutes for cooking.

15 to 20 minutes for preparation.

<u>Approximate nutritional information</u>

- *400 calories*

- *Fat: 18g*

- *33g of carbohydrates*

- *24g of protein*

<u>*Ingredients:*</u>

- *1 substantial tortilla wrap*

- *2 eggs*

- *1/4 cup chopped bell pepper, 1/4 cup diced onion*

- *1/4 cup of cheese, shredded*

- *25% of salsa*

- *Pepper and salt as desired*

- *Optional: avocado, spicy sauce, cubed gammon, fried bacon*

<u>*Makings:*</u>

- *Whisk the eggs with the salt and pepper in a small bowl.*

- *The onion and bell pepper should be cooked in a pan over medium heat until they are soft and just beginning to color.*

- *When the veggies are thoroughly cooked, add the eggs to the pan and scramble them along them.*

- *The tortilla should be soft and malleable after being warmed briefly in the microwave or on a griddle.*

- *Place the tortilla on a dish, then fill the center with the scrambled eggs and veggies.*

- *Add salsa, shredded cheese, and any other toppings you choose on top.*

- *The burrito is rolled up by folding the tortilla's sides inward and then securely wrapping it up from the bottom up.*

- *Serve right away.*

- *Note: Depending on the precise components you use and the serving size, the nutritional information may change.*

A breakfast burrito is a fantastic way to start the day with a healthy meal that is both delicious and filling. Feel free to be creative and make this dish your own by using your preferred vegetables, meats, and toppings!

BOWL OF CHEESE AND FRUIT, COTTAGE

This recipe makes enough for one serving.

5 minutes to prepare

0 minutes were spent cooking.

- *330 calories*
- *Protein 23g*
- *22 grams of carbs*
- *6g fiber, 12g fat*

Ingredients:

- *Cottage cheese, one cup*
- *1 cup of assorted fruits, such as bananas, apples, or berries*
- *Honey, two tablespoons*
- *(Optional) 1/4 cup chopped nuts*

Makings:

- *In a bowl, first, combine the cottage cheese and honey.*

- *Add your chosen fruit mixture and thoroughly combine.*

- *If used, top with chopped nuts.*

- *Enjoy your lovely dish of fruit and cottage cheese.*

HASH OF SWEET POTATO

Ingredients:

- *2 big sweet potatoes, diced after being peeled*
- *1 diced onion 1 diced red bell pepper*
- *1 diced green bell pepper*
- *Olive oil, two teaspoons*
- *Smoked paprika, 1 teaspoon*
- *One-half teaspoon of garlic powder*

- *4 eggs, salt & pepper to taste*

<u>*Makings:*</u>

- *Olive oil should be heated to a medium-high temperature in a big skillet.*

- *Add the diced sweet potatoes and simmer, turning periodically, for 10 to 15 minutes, or until they are soft but still somewhat crunchy.*

- *For a further 5-7 minutes, when the veggies are soft and caramelized, add the chopped onion and bell pepper.*

- *Add salt, pepper, garlic powder, and smoked paprika after stirring.*

- *Place four eggs over the hash in the same skillet and cover with a lid.*

- *Cook the eggs for a further 5-7 minutes, or until they are done to your preference.*

- *With the eggs on top, serve the hot sweet potato hash.*

FRUIT PANCAKE

Four servings may be made using this recipe.

Cooking time: The whole cooking process takes around 30 to 35 minutes.

Preparation time: It takes around 10-15 minutes to prepare.

- *267 calories*
- *Fat: 11g*
- *34g of carbohydrates*
- *8g protein*
- *6g of fiber*
- *10g sugar*

Ingredients:

- *One ripe banana*
- *1 egg*
- *All-purpose flour, half a cup*
- *A half-teaspoon of baking powder*
- *14 teaspoons of salt*
- *14 cups of milk*
- *Vegetable oil, 1 tablespoon*

- *Use a fork to mash the ripe banana in a medium mixing dish.*

- *After incorporating the egg, continue mixing.*

- *Once the mixture is smooth, add the flour, baking powder, salt, milk, and vegetable oil. Stir well.*

- *A nonstick skillet should be heated to medium.*

- *For each pancake, pour 1/4 cup of batter into the griddle.*

- *Cook the pancakes until golden brown, about 2-3 minutes on each side.*

- *With your preferred toppings, such as sliced bananas, honey, or maple syrup, serve the pancakes warm.*

CHAPTER 2

APPETIZER

AROMATIC ZUCCHINI CHIPS

This recipe yields around 2–3 servings.

15 minutes for preparation

20 to 25 minutes for cooking

Per-serving nutritional information:

- *153 calories*

- *Fat: 10g*

- *12g of carbohydrates*

- *2g of fiber*

- *5g protein*

Ingredients:

- *Two large courgette*

- *Panko breadcrumbs, half a cup*

- *Grated parmesan cheese, 1/4 cup*

- *12 teaspoons of garlic powder*

- *1/8 teaspoon of onion powder*

- *14 teaspoon salt*

- *Black pepper, 1/4 teaspoon*

- *2/TBS of olive oil*

- *Frying oil*

Makings:

- *For best results, line a baking sheet with parchment paper and preheat the oven to 425°F (218°C).*

- *Slice the zucchini into 1/4-inch-thick slices.*

- *Panko breadcrumbs, parmesan cheese, garlic powder, onion powder, salt, and black pepper should all be combined in a bowl.*

- *Each slice of zucchini is dipped in olive oil before being covered in the breadcrumb mixture. Place the coated slices on the baking sheet that has been prepared.*

- *To help the slices crisp up in the oven, sprinkle cooking spray over their tops.*

- *Slices should be baked for 20 to 25 minutes, turning them over halfway through, until crispy and golden brown.*

- *Before serving, take the zucchini chips out of the oven and let them cool for a while.*

SKEWERS FOR GREEK SALAD

Depending on the size of the skewers and the quantity of veggies used, this recipe yields 4-6 skewers.

15 minutes for preparation

5-7 minutes for cooking

Dietary information (per skewer):

- *160 calories*
- *14g total fat*
- *3g of saturated fat*
- *8 mg of cholesterol*

- *Salt: 320 mg*

- *7g of total carbs*

- *2g of dietary fiber*

- *4g sugars*

- *4g. protein*

Ingredients:

- *Cucumber, 1; Chop into pieces*

- *One red bell pepper, chopped*

- *One yellow bell pepper, chopped*

- *Cherry tomatoes in a pint*

- *Half a red onion, chopped*

- *Kalamata olives, 1/2 cup*

- *1/2 cup feta cheese crumbles*

- *Extra virgin olive oil, 1/4 cup*

- *Red wine vinegar, 2 teaspoons*

- *Oregano, dry, 1 teaspoon*

- *Black pepper with salt*

- *Skewers*

Makings:

- *To avoid scorching, soak the skewers in water for at least 30 minutes before using them.*

- *Combine the olive oil, red wine vinegar, oregano, salt, and black pepper in a large bowl.*

- *Toss the kalamata olives, red onion, cherry tomatoes, cucumber, bell peppers, and cherry tomatoes in the dressing in the bowl.*

- *You may arrange the feta cheese and veggies on the skewers as you prefer.*

- *The veggies should be browned and tender after grilling the skewers for 5 to 7 minutes over medium-high heat, flipping them over once or twice.*

- *Any leftover dressing should be poured over the skewers before serving.*

ROLL-UP EGGPLANTS

Size of serving: 4-6 persons

25 to 30 minutes for cooking

20 minutes for preparation

Per-serving nutritional information (based on 4 servings):

- *280 calories*

- *Fat: 12g*

- *23g of carbohydrates*

- *18g of protein*

- *7g of fiber*

Ingredients:

- *1 big aubergine, cut into 1/4-inch slices lengthwise.*

- *Marinara sauce, 1 cup*

- *Ricotta cheese, 1 cup*

- *Grated Parmesan cheese, 1/4 cup*

- *Shredded mozzarella cheese in a cup*

- *1 egg*

- *2 minced garlic cloves*

- *1/2 tsp. dried basil*

- *Pepper and salt as desired*

Makings:

- *Turn the oven on to 375°F.*

- *Combine the ricotta cheese, Parmesan cheese, garlic, egg, basil, salt, and pepper in a large bowl.*

- *On a baking sheet covered with parchment paper, spread out the eggplant slices.*

- *Each slice of aubergine should have a thin layer of cheese placed equally over it.*

- *Each aubergine slice should be rolled up before being placed seam-side down in a baking dish.*

- *The eggplant roll-ups should be covered with marinara sauce, then top with shredded mozzarella cheese.*

- *Bake the dish for 20 to 25 minutes, or until the cheese is melted and bubbling, covered with aluminum foil.*

- *Once the foil has been removed, bake the cheese for an additional 5 to 10 minutes, or until golden brown.*

- *Serving hot, please.*

VEGGIE AND HUMMUS PLATTER

Serving size: This recipe yields enough hummus for 6 to 8 people, and you may change the vegetables to suit your tastes.

Cooking time: This dish doesn't need any cooking time.

Time spent on preparation: 15 minutes or such.

Nutritional information:

The hummus and vegetable plate is a calorie-efficient, high-protein, high-fiber snack. The kind and amount of vegetables used may affect the precise nutritional value.

Ingredients:

- *1 can of washed and drained chickpeas*

- *Tahini, 14 cup*

- *2 minced garlic cloves*

- *Lemon juice, two teaspoons*

- *14 teaspoons of salt*

- *Olive oil, 1/4 cup*

- *Various veggies (such as carrots, cucumbers, bell peppers, etc.) for dipping*

Makings:

- *The chickpeas, tahini, garlic, lemon juice, and salt should be well combined in a food processor.*

- *Olive oil should be progressively added while the food processor is running until the mixture is creamy and well-mixed.*

- *If necessary, taste the hummus and adjust the spice.*

- *Place the hummus in the middle of a large dish after transferring it to a serving bowl.*

- *Around the hummus dish, arrange the veggies.*

- *Dispense and savor.*

The Hummus and Veggie Platter, in conclusion, is a tasty, nutritious, and simple-to-prepare appetizer that is ideal for any occasion. It's a fantastic method to increase your intake of vegetables while also wowing your visitors!

EDAMAME

Depending on your appetite, a portion of edamame should be between 1/2 and 1 cup.

Time spent cooking: It simply takes 5 to 10 minutes to cook one cup of edamame.

Edamame requires just a little amount of preparation time, which consists of washing and boiling the beans.

Nutritional information:

A serving of edamame (1/2 cup) provides 10% of your daily iron requirements, 120 calories, 11 grams of protein, and 5 grams of fiber. Additionally, they contain a lot of antioxidants and other healthy elements.

Ingredients:

- *1-2 cups of fresh or frozen edamame*

- *Salt (optional) Water*

<u>*Makings:*</u>

- *Edamame should be rinsed in a colander with cold running water.*

- *When using frozen edamame, defrost them overnight in the refrigerator or briefly submerge them in cold water.*

- *Bring water in a big saucepan to a boil. Add salt if desired.*

- *Depending on the texture required, add the edamame to the boiling water and cook for 5–10 minutes.*

- *To halt the cooking process, drain the edamame in a strainer and rinse under cold water.*

- *Add some more salt to the edamame before serving (optional).*

- *To sum up, preparing edamame at home is an easy and nutritious snack choice that everybody may enjoy.*

- *You may make a tasty and healthy snack that will satisfy your appetite and have many positive health effects with only a few easy steps.*

DEVILED AVOCADO EGGS

Servings: twelve

12 minutes for cooking

10 minutes for preparation

Dietary information (per serving):

- *74 calories*
- *Fat: 6g*
- *2g of carbohydrates*
- *3g. protein*

Ingredients:

- *6 hard-boiled eggs, divided in half and peeled*
- *1 pitted and mashed avocado*
- *2 tablespoons of mayo*
- *1/9 cup Dijon mustard*
- *A teaspoon of lime juice*
- *14 teaspoons of salt*
- *Black pepper, 1/8 teaspoon*
- *Paprika for adornment*

Makings:

- *The egg yolks should be taken out and put in a basin.*
- *Add the mayonnaise, Dijon mustard, lime juice, salt, and black pepper to the bowl along with the mashed avocado.*
- *The mixture should be well blended and creamy.*
- *Divide the mixture equally among the 12 halves before spooning it into the egg whites.*
- *For garnish, sprinkle with chopped cilantro and paprika.*
- *At least 30 minutes should pass before serving the deviled eggs from the refrigerator.*

Avocado deviled eggs are a tasty and healthy snack that is simple to prepare. They are a fantastic option for anybody seeking to eat healthily since they are packed with fiber, protein, and healthy fats. Try out this recipe and have fun!

RUBBERIZED MUSHROOMS

Serving Size: 4 individuals

20 to 25 minutes for cooking

10 minutes for preparation

Info about nutrition:

- *Kilocalories: 70*

- *4g of total fat*

- *1g of saturated fat*

- *5 mg of cholesterol*

- *Salt: 140 mg*

- *5g of total carbohydrates*

- *1g of dietary fiber*

- *2g sugars*

- *4g. protein*

Ingredients:

- *12 little mushrooms with stem out*
- *Breadcrumbs, half a cup*

- *Grated parmesan cheese, 1/4 cup*
- *14 cups of freshly chopped parsley*
- *Onion cut into 1/4 cup*
- *2 minced garlic cloves*
- *Olive oil, 1/4 cup*
- *Pepper and salt as desired*

Makings:

- *Turn the oven on to 375°F.*

- *Combine the breadcrumbs, parmesan cheese, parsley, onion, garlic, extra virgin olive oil, salt, and pepper in a medium bowl. Mix thoroughly.*

- *Place some of the breadcrumb mixtures into each mushroom cap. The mushrooms should be baked for 20 to 25 minutes, or until the caps are browned.*

- *Enjoy the hot-filled mushrooms after serving.*

Everyone may enjoy stuffed mushrooms, which are a flexible and healthful snack. Stuffed mushrooms are a great option whether you're looking for a fast and simple appetizer or a wholesome side dish.

Stuffed mushrooms are likely to become a staple in your kitchen because of their mouthwatering flavor and wholesome ingredients.

FRIED SUGAR POTATOES

This recipe is enough for two to three people as a side dish.

10 minutes for preparation

20 to 25 minutes for cooking

Nutrition information: Dietary fiber, potassium, and vitamins A and C are all abundant in sweet potato fries.

Approximately 280 calories, 5 grams of protein, 11 grams of fat, and 43 grams of carbs are included in each serving of this dish.

Ingredients:

- **2 substantial sweet potatoes**
- **Olive oil, 2 tablespoons**
- **Pepper and salt as desired**

Makings:

- **Set the oven to 425 °F.**

- **The sweet potatoes should be peeled and cut into fries of the same size.**

- **Add the olive oil to the sweet potato fries in a bowl. Toss to evenly coat the fries.**

- *To taste, add salt and pepper.*

- *Make sure the fries are spread out in a single layer and are not touching each other when you place them on a baking sheet covered with parchment paper.*

- *Bake the fries for 20 to 25 minutes or until crispy and browned. To achieve equal frying, flip the fries halfway through the cooking period.*

- *Serve hot after removing from the oven.*

PREMIUM SKEWERS

This recipe yields 16 skewers, which may be used as an appetizer or snack for 4 people.

15 minutes for preparation

5-7 minutes for cooking

Nutrition facts for a serving of four skewers:

- *215 calories*
- *14g total fat*
- *8g of saturated fat*
- *45 mg. cholesterol*
- *Salt: 342 mg*
- *10g of total carbs*
- *1g of dietary fiber*
- *8g sugars*
- *12g of protein*

Ingredients:

- *Cherry tomatoes, 16,*
- *16 balls of fresh mozzarella*

- *16 leaves of fresh basil*

- *Balsamic vinegar, 1/4 cup*

- *One tablespoon each of honey and olive oil*

- *pepper and salt as desired*

- *(16) skewers*

Makings:

To avoid burning them on the grill or in the oven, start by soaking the skewers in water for at least 30 minutes.

Until all the skewers are put together, alternate threading one cherry tomato, one mozzarella ball, and one basil leaf onto each skewer.

Balsamic vinegar and honey should be combined in a small saucepan, and they should be heated over medium heat while being regularly stirred until the liquid has thickened and reduced by half. It ought to should take five to seven minutes.

Set the temperature of your oven or grill to medium-high. Olive oil should be used to coat the skewers before seasoning with salt and pepper.

To melt the cheese and slightly sear the tomatoes, grill or bake the skewers for approximately 5 minutes, rotating them halfway through.

After removing the skewers from the fire, cover them with the balsamic glaze. Serve right away.

CUCUMBER MUGS

Size of serving: 4-6 persons

0 minutes were spent cooking.

15 minutes for preparation

- *31 calories*
- *0.5g total fat*
- *6g of total carbs*
- *2g protein*
- *1g of fiber*

Ingredients:

- *2 substantial cukes*
- *4 oz. softened cream cheese*
- *1/4 cup red bell peppers, chopped*
- *1/4 cup red onion, chopped*
- *1 teaspoon freshly chopped dill*
- *Pepper and salt as desired*

Makings:

- *Cut the ends off the cucumbers after washing. Cucumbers should be cut into 1-inch chunks.*

- *Scoop off the seeds from the center of each cucumber slice, leaving a thin rim around the edge, using a tiny spoon or melon baller.*

- *Mix the cream cheese, diced red bell pepper, diced red onion, salt, pepper, and chopped dill in a medium bowl.*

- *Put a tiny amount of the cream cheese mixture into each cucumber cup.*
- *Before serving, place the cucumber cups in the refrigerator to chill for at least 30 minutes.*

A low-calorie, high-fiber snack like cucumber cups is ideal for anybody controlling their weight. Additionally, they are an excellent source of potassium and vitamin C. To make a range of delectable appetizers, experiment with various fillings, such as hummus, tuna salad, or guacamole. Enjoy

CHAPTER 3

BEEF

SKEWERS OF BEEF GRILLED WITH VEGETABLES

Serving size nutrition facts:

- *377 calories*
- *22g total fat*
- *5g of saturated fat*
- *90 mg cholesterol*
- *Salt: 151 mg*
- *10g of total carbs*
- *2g of dietary fiber*

- *Sucrose: 6g*

- *34g of protein*

<u>*Ingredients:*</u>

- *Beef sirloin weighing 1 lb., sliced into 1-inch chunks*

- *One seeded red bell pepper, diced into 1-inch pieces.*

- *1 seeded and cut into 1-inch pieces yellow bell pepper*

- *Cut one red onion into 1-inch slices.*

- *Cut one zucchini into 1-inch slices.*

- *Olive oil, 1/4 cup*

- *Balsamic vinegar, two teaspoons*

- *2 minced garlic cloves*

- *Oregano, dry, 1 teaspoon*

- *Pepper and salt as desired*

- *4–6 skewers, soaking for at least 30 minutes in water*

- *Heat your grill to a moderately hot setting.*

- *Combine the olive oil, balsamic vinegar, garlic, oregano, salt, and pepper in a small bowl.*

- *On the skewers, arrange the meat, bell peppers, onion, and zucchini.*

- *Apply the marinade on the skewers.*

- *As the steak cooks to the desired degree of doneness, flip the skewers every 10 to 12 minutes on the grill.*

- *Serve the skewers hot, along with a side salad or rice, and your preferred dipping sauce.*

BEEF STEW IN SLOW COOKER WITH LOW-SODIUM BROTH

Portion size

There are 6 servings in this recipe.

Time Required for Cooking: The cooking process takes around 8 hours on low heat or 4 hours on high heat.

Preparation Time: It takes around 20 minutes to prepare.

Nutritional Information: There are around 330 calories, 18 grams of fat, 23 grams of carbs, 20 grams of protein, and 460 milligrams of sodium in each serving of this slow-cooker beef stew.

- *Cubed beef stew meat weighing 2 pounds, plus 1/4 cup of all-purpose flour*
- *1 salt shaker*
- *Black pepper, half a teaspoon*
- *Olive oil, two teaspoons*
- *1 diced onion, 3 minced garlic cloves*
- *4 cups of beef broth low in salt*
- *One water cup*
- *One tablespoon of dried thyme*
- *1 teaspoon of rosemary, dry*
- *1 cup of frozen peas, 3 big carrots, 3 celery stalks, and 3 medium potatoes, peeled and cubed*
- *Fresh parsley garnish, chopped (optional)*

Makings:

- *Combine the flour, salt, and pepper in a bowl. Shake off any extra flour as you coat the beef stew meat.*

- *Olive oil should be heated to a medium-high temperature in a big skillet. About 5 minutes after adding the beef, brown both sides of the meat.*

- *Enter the slow cooker with the meat.*

- *The onion and garlic should be added to the same pan and cooked for approximately 3 minutes, until tender. To the slow cooker, add the onion and garlic.*

- *To the slow cooker, add the beef broth, water, thyme, and rosemary. To blend, stir.*

- *Stir the potatoes, celery, and carrots after adding them to the slow cooker.*

- *Cook the meat and veggies undercover for 8 hours on low or 4 hours on high, or until they are soft.*

- *Add the frozen peas and toss to incorporate during the last 15 minutes of simmering.*

- *If desired, top the hot beef stew with fresh parsley that has been chopped.*

- *Enjoy your flavorful and nutritious Slow Cooker Low Sodium Beef Stew.*

LOW-SODIUM SOY SAUCE IN A STIR-FRY WITH BEEF AND BROCCOLI

Servings: four

10 minutes for preparation

Time to cook: 10 minutes

- *256 calories*
- *12g total fat*
- *3g of saturated fat*
- *68mg of cholesterol*
- *Salt: 398 mg*
- *9g of total carbohydrates*
- *2g of dietary fiber*
- *2g sugar*
- *27g of protein*

Ingredients:

- *1 pound of finely cut against the grain flank steak*
- *broccoli florets, 3 cups*
- *3 minced garlic cloves*

* *Corn flour, one tablespoon*
* *Low-sodium soy sauce, 14 cup*
* *14 cups of water*
* *Vegetable oil, 1 tablespoon*
* *Pepper and salt as desired*

Makings:

* *Combine the corn flour, soy sauce, and water in a small bowl. Place aside.*

* *In a large skillet or wok, heat the oil over medium-high heat.*
* *30 seconds later, add the garlic and sauté until fragrant.*

* *Add the meat and stir-fry for 3–4 minutes, or until browned.*

- *When the broccoli is soft but still crisp, add the broccoli and stir-fry for an additional two to three minutes.*

- *When the sauce has thickened, approximately 1-2 minutes, pour the soy sauce mixture over the meat and broccoli while continuously stirring.*

- *To taste, add salt and pepper to the food.*

- *Serve hot with noodles or rice.*

SOUP OF BEEF AND VEGETABLES WITHOUT ADDING SALT

Serving Size: There are 4-6 servings in this dish.

Cooking time: Preparing and cooking this soup takes around 1 hour and 15 minutes.

Preparation: This dish requires around 15 minutes of preparation.

Information about diet:

- *233 calories*
- *Fat: 6g*
- *2g of saturated fat*
- *70 mg. cholesterol*
- *Salt: 84 mg*
- *17g of carbohydrates*
- *3g of fiber*
-
- *4g sugar*
- *27g of protein*

Ingredients:

1 pound of bite-sized chunks of beef stew meat

2 cups water and 2 cups low-sodium beef broth

One onion, minced; two garlic cloves; two carrots; two celery stalks; two potatoes; one cup of frozen green beans.

One tablespoon of dried thyme

Black pepper, half a teaspoon

Makings:

- *The steak should be well-browned over medium-high heat until it is no longer pink. Remove any extra fat.*

- *When the onion is transparent, add it to the stew along with the garlic.*

- *To the saucepan, add the beef broth, water, celery, carrots, potatoes, green beans, thyme, pepper, and bay leaf. To blend, stir.*

- *The soup should be brought to a boil, then simmer for an hour, or until the vegetables are fork-tender and the meat is well cooked.*

- *Before serving, take the bay leaf out.*

LOW SODIUM BUTTER-MADE PAN-SEARED BEEF TENDERLOIN WITH HERB BUTTER

Each steak in this dish weighs 4 ounces and feeds four people.

10 minutes for preparation

10 to 12 minutes for cooking

Dietary information (per serving):

- *292 calories*

- *Fat: 15g*

- *31g of protein*

- *0g of carbohydrates*

- *0g of fiber*

- *Salt: 235 mg*

Ingredients:

- *4 beef tenderloin steaks, each weighing 4 oz.*

- *Black pepper and 1/4 teaspoon each of salt*

- *Butter low in sodium, 2 teaspoons*

- *1 tablespoon of fresh herbs, such as parsley, thyme, and rosemary, chopped*

Makings:

- *Set the oven to 400 °F.*

- *On both sides, season the beef tenderloin steaks with salt and black pepper.*

- *A big skillet should be heated up extremely hot over high heat. The steaks should be added and seared for two to three minutes on each side, or until browned and caramelized.*

- *For medium-rare, place the pan in the preheated oven and cook the steaks for 5-7 minutes, or until they are cooked to your preference.*

- *Transfer the steaks to a dish after taking the pan out of the oven. Put a foil tent over them and let those five to ten minutes to rest.*

- *Melt the low-sodium butter in a small saucepan over medium heat. Stir in the freshly chopped herbs after adding them.*

- *Slice the steaks and place the herb butter on top before serving.*

FISH

SALMON WITH LEMON HERB BAKED

This dish makes plenty for four people to eat.

Cooking time: The cooking process takes 20 to 25 minutes.

Preparation time: It takes around 10-15 minutes to prepare.

Nutrition information: A serving of baked lemon herb salmon has around 300 calories, 35 grams of protein, and 10 grams of fat.

Ingredients:

- *4 skin-on salmon fillets*
- *2/TBS of olive oil*
- *2 tablespoons lemon juice, fresh*
- *1 teaspoon Dijon mustard*
- *1 tablespoon of honey*
- *Dry thyme, 1 teaspoon*
- *1 teaspoon dried rosemary*
- *12 teaspoons of garlic powder*
- *To taste, add salt and black pepper.*
- *Fresh parsley and lemon wedges are used as a garnish.*

Makings:

- *Set the oven's temperature to 400°F (200°C). Use parchment paper to cover a baking sheet.*

- *Olive oil, lemon juice, Dijon mustard, honey, dried thyme, dried rosemary, garlic powder, salt, and black pepper should all be combined in a small bowl.*

- *Place the salmon fillets on the prepared baking sheet skin side down.*

- *Make careful to properly coat the salmon fillets with the lemon-herb mixture.*

- *The salmon fillets should be cooked through and flaky after 20 to 25 minutes in the oven.*

- *After taking the salmon out of the oven, give it some time to rest.*

- *With lemon wedges and fresh parsley for garnish, serve the salmon fillets.*

- *Enjoy your tasty and nutritious baked salmon with lemon and herbs.*

TUNA STEAK GRILLED

10 minutes for preparation
6 to 8 minutes for cooking

Nutrition information:

- *Size of Serving: 1 tuna steak*
- *240 calories*
- *11g total fat*
- *2g of saturated fat*
- *65mg of cholesterol*

- *Salt: 640 mg*

- *1 g of carbohydrates overall*

- *0g of dietary fiber*

- *34g of protein*

Ingredients:

- *4 6 ounce apiece tuna steaks*

- *Olive oil, two teaspoons*

- *One teaspoon of lemon juice*

- *1 salt shaker*

- *Black pepper, half a teaspoon*

- *2 minced garlic cloves*

- *1/4 teaspoon optional red pepper flakes*

Makings:

- *Heat your grill to a moderately hot setting.*

- *Mix the olive oil, lemon juice, salt, black pepper, minced garlic, and red pepper flakes (if using) in a small bowl.*

- *The marinade should be applied on both sides of the tuna steaks.*

- *Depending on the thickness of the steak, place the tuna steaks on the hot grill and cook for 2 to 3 minutes on each side.*

- *When the tuna steaks are done to your preference, take them from the grill and give them a few minutes to rest before serving.*

In conclusion, grilled tuna steak is a quick and wholesome supper that takes less than 30 minutes to make. It's a fantastic choice for a nutritious midweek supper or a post-workout meal due to its high protein and nutritional content.

SWORDFISH BROILED WITH TOMATO AND BASIL

10 minutes for preparation

15 to 20 minutes for cooking

Calorie information per serving:

- *375 calories*

- *20g total fat*

- *3g of saturated fat*

- *80 mg cholesterol*

- *Salt: 190 mg*

- *5g of total carbs*

- *1g of dietary fiber*

- *3g sugars*

- *44g of protein*

Ingredients:

- *4 swordfish steaks, each weighing around 6 ounces*
- *2 big, chopped tomatoes*
- *14 cups finely minced fresh basil*
- *Olive oil, 1/4 cup*
- *2 minced garlic cloves*
- *Pepper and salt*

<u>*Makings:*</u>

- *Set the grill to high.*

- *Combine the minced garlic, basil, olive oil, and chopped tomatoes in a small bowl. To taste, add salt and pepper to the food.*
- *On both sides, season the swordfish steaks with salt and pepper.*

- *Swordfish steaks should be broiled until cooked through and gently browned, which takes approximately 5-7 minutes on each side.*

- *Serve the tomato and basil combination on top of each swordfish steak.*

- *One swordfish steak with tomatoes and basil per serving.*

DOLPHIN POACHED WITH VEGETABLES

This dish yields enough food for four persons.

Cooking Time: This meal takes around 20 minutes to prepare.

Preparation Time: This dish requires around 10 minutes of preparation.

Nutrition information: 242 calories, 5g of fat, 14g of carbs, 36g of protein, and 5g of fiber.

Ingredients:

- *4 fillets of cod*
- *White wine, half a cup*
- *2 glasses of water*
- *Olive oil, 2 tablespoons*
- *1 sliced red pepper, 2 minced garlic cloves, 2 chopped carrots, 1 sliced onion, and 1 sliced zucchini*
- *To taste, add salt and pepper.*

Makings:

- *Bring the white wine and water to a boil in a big saucepan.*

- *Then turn down the heat to a simmer and add the fish fillets.*

- *Cook the fish underneath for 5–7 minutes, or until it is well done.*

- *Olive oil should be heated in a separate pan over medium heat.*

- *When the onion is tender and transparent, add the garlic and onion.*

- *Add the zucchini, red pepper, celery, carrots, and celery to the pan. Cook for 5-7 minutes, or until the veggies are soft.*

- *Add salt and pepper to taste and season the veggies.*

- *On top of the prepared veggies, plate the poached cod fillets.*

TILAPIA PAN-FRIED WITH LEMON AND THYME

Servings: two

10 minutes for preparation

Time to Cook: 10 minutes

Per-serving nutritional information:

- *215 calories*
- *Fat: 11g*
- *2g of carbohydrates*

- *28g of protein*
- *Salt: 106 mg*

<u>*Ingredients:*</u>

- *2 fillets of tilapia*
- *1 tablespoon of olive oil*
- *2 chopped garlic cloves, 1 sliced lemon, and 4-5 fresh thyme sprigs*
- *Pepper and salt as desired*

<u>*Makings:*</u>

- *In a large skillet over medium-high heat, warm the olive oil.*

- *Salt and pepper the tilapia fillets on both sides.*

- *When the oil in the pan is heated, add the minced garlic and cook until fragrant, about 1 minute.*

- *The tilapia fillets should be added to the pan and cooked for 3–4 minutes on each side or until golden and fully done.*

- *Slices of lemon and fresh thyme should be added to the skillet. Cook for an additional 1-2 minutes, or until the lemon is just beginning to caramelize.*

- *The fish should be served with lemon slices and thyme sprigs on top once the pan has been taken from the heat.*

This pan-fried tilapia with lemon and thyme is low in carbs, high in protein, and healthy fats. You may easily alter it by using your preferred veggies or a side salad. Enjoy!

CHAPTER 4

VEGETARIAN AND VEGAN RECIPES

LEMON SOUP

Size of servings: 4-6

10 minutes for preparation

30 minutes for cooking

Dietary information (per serving):

- *259 calories*

- *16 g of protein*
- *Fat: 3 g*

- *44 g of carbohydrates*

- *16 g of fiber*

Ingredients:

- *1 cup of washed and drained lentils*
- *One sliced onion*
- *3 minced garlic cloves*
- *Two sliced carrots and two chopped celery stalks*
- *Olive oil, 1 tbsp.*
- *4 cups of veggie broth*

- *1 tomato-diced can*

- *1 teaspoon each of ground cumin and coriander*

- *Smoked paprika, 1 teaspoon*

- *To taste, add salt and pepper.*

- *Chopped fresh parsley for a garnish*

Makings:

- *Olive oil is heated over medium heat in a big saucepan. For approximately 3 minutes, add the onion and garlic and sauté until tender.*

- *For a further 3-5 minutes, or until the veggies are just beginning to soften, add the carrots and celery.*

- *Cumin, coriander, smoked paprika, chopped tomatoes, lentils, vegetable broth, salt, and pepper should all be added to the saucepan. To blend, thoroughly stir.*

- *Heat should be turned down once the soup comes to a boil. For 20 to 25 minutes, or until the lentils are soft, cover and simmer the mixture.*

- *Pour the soup into a blender or use an immersion blender to purée it until smooth.*

- *If necessary, taste and adjust the spices. Serve hot with fresh parsley as a garnish.*

- *On a cold day, indulge in this hearty and soothing lentil soup. It's a fantastic lunch or supper option, and leftovers keep for up to 5 days in the refrigerator.*

SALAD DE QUINOA

Serving size nutrition facts:

- *340 calories*

- *Fat: 18g*

- *2.5g of saturated fat*
- *0 mg of cholesterol*

- *20 milligrams of sodium*

- *39g of carbohydrates*

- *6g of fiber*

- *3g of sugar*

- *7g protein*

Servings: four

15 minutes for preparation

20 minutes for cooking

<u>*Ingredients:*</u>

- *Quinoa, one cup*
- *2-cups of water*
- *1 diced red bell pepper 1 diced cucumber*
- *Chopped red onion, half*
- *Fresh cilantro and parsley, each cut into a quarter cup*
- *14 cups finely minced fresh mint*
- *Olive oil, 1/4 cup*
- *Lemon juice, 1/4 cup*
- *Pepper and salt as desired*

<u>*Makings:*</u>

- *Drain the quinoa after rinsing it in a sieve with fine mesh.*

- *Bring the quinoa and water to a boil in a medium saucepan.*

- *Once the water has been absorbed and the quinoa is soft, turn the heat down to low and continue to simmer for 15 to 20 minutes.*

- *Quinoa should be taken off the heat and given some time to cool.*

- *The cooked quinoa, red bell pepper, cucumber, red onion, parsley, cilantro, and mint should all be combined in a big dish.*

- *Mix the olive oil, lemon juice, salt, and pepper in a small bowl. Toss the quinoa mixture with the dressing after pouring it over it.*

- *The quinoa salad may be served cold or warm.*

SWEET POTATO BAKED

There are 4 servings in this recipe.

Five minutes to prepare.

45 to 60 minutes for cooking.

Dietary information (per serving):

- *161 calories*
- *Fat: 5g*

- *27g of carbohydrates*

- *4g of fiber*

- *2g protein*

- *438% DV of vitamin A*

- *4% DV of vitamin C*

- *4% DV for calcium*

- *Fe: 4% DV*

Ingredients:

- *4 large sweet potatoes*

- *Olive oil, two teaspoons*

- *To taste, add salt and pepper.*

- *Butter, cinnamon, brown sugar, and marshmallows are optional toppings.*

Makings:

- *Turn on the oven to 400 °F (200 °C).*

- *Cleanse the sweet potatoes well with running water, then pat them dry.*

- *Each potato should have multiple fork pricks on both sides to enable steam to escape during baking.*
- *Olive oil should be applied to each potato, and salt and pepper should be used liberally.*

- *Put the sweet potatoes on a baking sheet that has been coated with aluminum foil or parchment paper.*

- *Bake the sweet potatoes for 45 to 60 minutes, or until they can easily be punctured with a fork. The thickness and size of your potatoes will determine the precise cooking time.*

- *Before serving, take the sweet potatoes out of the oven and allow them cool for a while.*

- *Make a slit on the top of each potato, then top with your preferred ingredients, such as marshmallows, butter, cinnamon, or brown sugar.*

STIR-FRIES WITH VEGETABLES

Servings: 2 to 3

15 to 20 minutes for cooking

10 minutes for preparation

Information about diet:

- *150 calories*
- *5g protein*
- *19g of carbohydrates*
- *Fat: 7g*

- *6g of fiber*
- *Sucrose: 7g*
- *Salt: 430 mg*

<u>*Ingredients:*</u>

- *Vegetable oil, two teaspoons*
- *1 minced garlic clove*
- *Sliced half an onion, cut half a bell pepper*
- *Broccoli florets, half a cup*
- *Sliced mushrooms in a cup*
- *Sliced carrots, one*
- *0.5 teaspoons of salt*
- *Black pepper, 1/4 teaspoon*
- *A serving of soy sauce*
- *50 ml of sesame oil*
- *Corn flour, one tablespoon*
- *1/4 cup water or vegetable broth*

<u>*Makings:*</u>

- *In a wok or large skillet, heat the vegetable oil over medium-high heat.*

- *Stir-fry the onion slices and minced garlic for one to two minutes, or until aromatic.*

- *Add the sliced carrot, sliced mushrooms, sliced bell pepper, and florets of broccoli and stir-fry for 3 to 4 minutes, or until the veggies are crisp-tender.*

- *Add the soy sauce and sesame oil after seasoning the veggies with salt and black pepper. Stir and cook for one minuter.*

- *Mix the corn flour and water or vegetable broth in a small basin, then pour the mixture into the pan. Stir-*

fry the veggies for 1-2 minutes, or until they are covered in sauce and it has thickened.

- *If desired, top the hot vegetable stir-fry with sesame seeds or sliced green onions.*

- *Enjoy your wonderful and nutritious stir-fry of vegetables.*

CURRY OF CHICKPEAS

This recipe makes enough for four people to eat it.

Cooking Time: This meal takes around 30 minutes to prepare.

Preparation Time: This dish requires roughly 10 minutes of preparation.

<u>*Nutritional data:*</u> This chickpea curry has around 250 calories per serving, 8 grams of protein, and 9 grams of fiber.

<u>*Ingredients:*</u>

- *1 can of washed and drained chickpeas*
- *1 diced onion, 2 minced garlic cloves*
- *Olive oil, 1 tbsp.*
- *1 teaspoon each of ground cumin and coriander*
- *1 teaspoon of turmeric, ground*
- *1/8 teaspoon cinnamon powder*
- *1/four teaspoon cayenne*
- *1 tomato-diced can*
- *A half-cup of vegetable broth*
- *To taste, add salt and pepper.*
- *For garnish: fresh cilantro*

<u>*Makings:*</u>

- *Over medium heat, warm the olive oil in a big saucepan.*

- *Sauté the garlic and onion together for two to three minutes, or until the onion is transparent.*

- *Stir together the cumin, coriander, turmeric, cinnamon, and cayenne pepper in the saucepan.*

- *Chickpeas, diced tomatoes, and vegetable broth should all be added to the saucepan. To taste, add salt and pepper to the food.*

- *The mixture should be brought to a boil, then simmer for 20 to 25 minutes, or until the sauce has thickened and the chickpeas are cooked through.*

- *Hot chickpea curry should be served with fresh cilantro on top.*

- *This recipe for chickpea curry is simple to prepare, tasty, and healthful. It's ideal for supper with friends and family or a simple midweek meal.*

CHAPTER 5

RECIPES FOR SALAD AND SANDWICHES

CUCUMBER AND TOMATO SALAD

10 minutes for preparation

0 minutes were spent cooking.

Duration: ten minutes

<u>*Serving size nutrition facts:*</u>

- *80 calories*
- *7g of total fat*
- *1g of saturated fat*
- *0 mg of cholesterol*
- *Salt: 75 mg*
- *4g of total carbohydrates*
- *1g of dietary fiber*
- *2g sugars*
- *1 g of protein*

<u>*Ingredients:*</u>

- *2 tablespoons olive oil, 2 big tomatoes, 1 large cucumber, 1/4 red onion, thinly sliced, and 1/4 cup fresh parsley, chopped*
- *1/fourth cup red wine vinegar*
- *Pepper and salt as desired*

Makings:

- *Combine the red onion, cucumber, and tomato slices in a big bowl.*

- *Whisk the olive oil, red wine vinegar, salt, and pepper in a separate small bowl.*

- *The dressing should be poured over the veggies, then mixed.*

- *Add the parsley and gently mix once more.*

* *Serve right away or keep chilled until you're ready to.*

Cucumbers and tomatoes both provide a lot of fiber and few calories, so this salad is a fantastic choice for anybody trying to eat healthily. Olive oil adds heart-healthy lipids, while red wine vinegar offers a tart flavor that goes well with the tomatoes' sweetness and the cucumbers' crispness. Enjoy this salad as a side dish or turn it into a whole dinner by adding some grilled chicken or prawns.

SALAD OF SPINACH AND BERRIES

There are 4 servings in this recipe.

10 minutes for preparation
0 minutes were spent cooking.

- *174 calories*
- *10g total fat*
- *1g of saturated fat*
- *0 mg of cholesterol*
- *Salt: 15 mg*
- *22g of total carbohydrates*
- *6g of dietary fiber*
- *14g sugars*
- *4g. protein*

Ingredients:

- *Fresh spinach, 5 oz.*
- *1 cup sliced strawberries*
- *Blueberries, 1 cup*
- *Chopped pecans, 1/4 cup*

- *Balsamic vinegar, 2 tbsp.*

- *1 tablespoon of honey*

- *Extra virgin olive oil, 1/4 cup*

- *Pepper and salt as desired*

Makings:

- *Rinse the spinach and use paper towels to wipe it dry.*

- *Combine the spinach, strawberries, blueberries, and pecans in a big bowl.*

- *Combine the balsamic vinegar, honey, and extra virgin olive oil in a small bowl.*

- *Toss the salad with the dressing after pouring it over it.*

- *To taste, add salt and pepper to the food.*

- *Serve right away or keep chilled until you're ready to.*

A delicious way to increase your intake of fruits and veggies is with this spinach and berry salad. You may have a filling and healthy lunch in a matter of minutes thanks to its quick preparation and delectable flavor.

A SALAD OF TUNA AND GREEN BEANS

This dish yields enough food for four persons.

15 minutes for preparation

10 minutes for cooking

Nutrition information:

- *240 calories*
- *Fat: 11g*

- *10g of carbohydrates*
- *27g of protein*
- *3g of fiber*
- *Salt: 410 mg*

Ingredients:

- *12 ounces of flaked and drained canned tuna*
- *trimming and chopping 8 ounces of green beans into bite-sized portions*
- *14 cups coarsely chopped red onion*
- *2 tablespoons chopped fresh parsley*
- *1.5 tbsp. lemon juice*
- *Extra virgin olive oil, 1/4 cup*
- *1-tablespoon Dijon mustard*
- *1 minced garlic clove*
- *Pepper and salt as desired*

Makings:

- *Boil some salted water in a pot. Green beans should be added and cooked for 3 to 4 minutes, or until crisp and tender. To halt the cooking process, drain the green beans and give them a cold water rinse.*

- *Green beans, red onion, parsley, and tuna that have been drained and flaked should all be combined in a big dish.*

- *Lemon juice, olive oil, Dijon mustard, garlic, salt, and pepper should all be well mixed in a small bowl.*

- *After adding the dressing, gently toss the tuna and green bean combination to coat.*

- *Taste-test the spices and serve cold.*

- *All in all, making this tuna salad with green beans is a simple, delectable supper. It is the ideal choice for individuals who want a fast and wholesome dinner.*

APPLE AND CHICKEN SALAD

Calorie information per serving:

- *366 calories*
- *26g of protein*
- *32g of carbohydrates*
- *Fat: 15g*
- *2g of saturated fat*
- *65mg of cholesterol*
- *Salt: 213 mg*
- *5g of fiber*
- *23g of sugar*

Take pleasure in your tasty and nutritious chicken and apple salad.

Servings: four

15 minutes for preparation
15 minutes for cooking

Ingredients:

- *2 skinless, boneless breasts of chicken*
- *Diced from two medium apples*
- *Dried cranberries in a half-cup*
- *A half-cup of chopped pecans*
- *Greek yogurt, plain, in 1/2 cup*
- *Mayonnaise, 1/4 cup*
- *Honey, two tablespoons*
- *1 teaspoon vinegar made from apple cider*
- *To taste, add salt and pepper.*

- *Lettuce greens*

Makings:

- *Turn the oven on to 375°F. The chicken breasts are put on a baking pan after being salt and pepper-seasoned. Bake for fifteen minutes, or until well done. Slice into bite-sized pieces after allowing to cool.*

- *Combine the diced apples, dried cranberries, pecans, and chicken in a large bowl.*

- *To prepare the dressing, combine the Greek yogurt, mayonnaise, honey, apple cider vinegar, salt, and pepper in a separate bowl.*

- *Then, coat the chicken and apple mixture with the dressing by pouring it over top.*

- *A bed of salad greens should be used to serve the chicken and apple salad.*

SALAD WITH BEETS AND FETA

This recipe makes enough for four people to eat it.

Cooking Time: Preparing this meal takes around one hour.

Preparation Time: This dish requires around 20 minutes of preparation time.

Nutritional Information:

- *170 calories*
- *9g total fat*

- *4g of saturated fat*
- *20 mg cholesterol*
- *Salt: 450 mg*
- *17g of total carbohydrates*
- *3g of dietary fiber*
- *14g sugar*
- *7g protein*

Ingredients:

- *Cut and cleaned four medium-sized beets*
- *1/2 cup feta cheese crumbles*
- *Chopped walnuts, 1/4 cup*
- *Balsamic vinegar, 2 tablespoons*
- *2 tablespoons of olive oil*
- *Pepper and salt as desired*
- *Greens like a rocket or a mix*

Makings:

- *Turn the oven on to 375°F.*

- *Each beet is covered in aluminum foil before being placed on a baking pan. Cook for 45 to 50 minutes, or until tender, in the oven.*

- *The beets should be taken out of the oven, unwrapped, and allowed to cool completely before handling. The beets should be skinless before being cut into tiny circles.*

- *To create the dressing, combine the olive oil and balsamic vinegar in a large basin.*

- *Sliced beets should be added to the dressing-filled dish and coated.*

- *Then, carefully mix in the feta cheese that has been crumbled and the chopped walnuts.*

- *To taste, add salt and pepper to the food.*

- *Over a bed of rockets or mixed greens, plate the salad.*

- *Take pleasure in your savory and nourishing beetroot and feta salad.*

MENU FOR SANDWICHES

CHICKEN SANDWICH, GRILLED

Size of serving: 1 sandwich

15 to 20 minutes for cooking

10 minutes for preparation

Dietary information (per serving):

- *400 calories*

- *Fat: 15g*

- *30g of carbohydrates*

- *35g of protein*

Ingredients:

- *1 skinless, boneless breast of chicken*

- *Olive oil, 1 tbsp.*

- *1/4 teaspoon black pepper and 1/2 teaspoon salt*

- *Two pieces of whole grain bread*

- *A serving of mayonnaise*

- *A single tomato slice*

- *1 lettuce leaf*

Makings:

- *Set the heat to medium-high on the grill or grill pan.*

- *Olive oil should be used to coat the chicken breast before adding salt and pepper.*

- *Grilled chicken breasts should be cooked for 6 to 8 minutes on each side, or until they reach an internal temperature of 165°F.*

- *Chicken should be taken from the grill and given five minutes to rest.*

- *Bread pieces are toasted before being smeared with mayonnaise on one side.*

- *One chicken breast should be placed on one piece of bread, followed by a slice of lettuce and tomato.*

- *Serve warm.*

You may marinate the chicken breast in your preferred marinade before grilling the sandwich to enhance the flavor. Additionally, you may add other toppings like cheddar, bacon, or avocado. Depending on the additional toppings, adjust the nutritional information appropriately.

SANDWICH WITH EGG SALAD

This recipe feeds two to three people.

10 minutes for cooking

10 minutes for preparation

Information about diet:

- *414 calories*
- *26g total fat*

- *6g of saturated fat*

- *383 mg of cholesterol*

- *Salt: 675 mg*

- *27g of total carbohydrates*

- *2g of dietary fiber*

- *5g of total sugars*

- *18g of protein*

Ingredients:

- *6 eggs*

- *Mayonnaise, 1/4 cup*

- *1 teaspoon Dijon mustard 2 teaspoons fresh parsley, chopped*

- *1 tablespoon freshly chopped chives*

- *Black pepper and 1/4 teaspoon each of salt*

- *Six pieces of bread*

- *Lettuce, if desired*

- *First, cook the eggs. Put the eggs in a saucepan and add cold water to cover them. Bring to a boil, then simmer for 8 to 10 minutes.*

- *The eggs should then be taken out of the saucepan and dropped into a dish of cold water to chill.*

- *Peel and slice the cooled eggs into little pieces when they have cooled.*

- *Combine the mayonnaise, Dijon mustard, parsley, chives, salt, and pepper in a separate bowl. Add the chopped eggs and stir everything together well.*

- *After toasting the bread pieces, put the sandwich together. One piece of bread should first have a layer of lettuce (if used), followed by egg salad. Add the second piece of bread on top.*

- *Serve the sandwich by cutting it in half.*

- *Enjoy your tasty sandwich with egg salad.*

SANDWICH WITH TUNA SALAD

Nutritional data: This tuna salad sandwich has 440 calories, 28g of fat, 22g of carbs, and 24g of protein per serving. This dish has a healthy amount of protein, and you may increase its nutritional value by using whole-grain bread and using extra veggies, such as bell pepper or cucumber.

Ingredients:

- *Two drained tuna cans*
- *Mayonnaise, half a cup*
- *14 cups of celery, chopped*

- *Red onion, diced, to equal 1/4 cup; fresh parsley, chopped to equal 2 tbsps.*

- *Lemon juice, 1 tablespoon*

- *Pepper and salt as desired*

- *Eight pieces of bread*

- *Sliced tomato and lettuce leaves as a garnish (optional)*

Makings:

- *Tuna that has been drained, mayonnaise, celery, red onion, parsley, lemon juice, salt, and pepper should all be combined in a mixing dish. All components should be well combined.*

- *The bread pieces should be gently browned after being toasted in a toaster or under the grill.*

- *Spread the tuna salad mixture equally over the four pieces of bread.*

- *The remaining pieces of bread should be placed on top of each sandwich after adding a lettuce leaf and a tomato slice (if using).*

- *Serve each sandwich cut in half.*

A VEGAN SANDWICH

Size of serving: 1 sandwich

10 minutes for preparation

Cooking period: 0

Information about diet:

- *398 calories*

- *Fat: 16g*

- *54g of carbohydrates*

- *14g of protein*

- *12g of fiber*

- *Salt: 459 mg*

Ingredients:

- *2 pieces of whole grain bread, or your favorite kind.*

- *Mashed avocado, half*

- *14 cups of hummus*

- *Carrots, shredded, 14 cup*

- *14 cups of cucumber slices*

- *1/4 cup of tomato slices*

- *Sliced bell pepper, 1/4 cup*

- *14 cups of red onion slices*

- *Several spinach leaves*

- *Pepper and salt as desired*

- *Toasted bread should be as crunchy as you want.*
- *On one piece of bread, spread mashed avocado; on the other, hummus.*

- *On one piece of bread, arrange the spinach, red onion, bell pepper, cucumber, tomato, and shredded carrots.*

- *Add pepper and salt to taste.*

- *With the second piece of bread, assemble the sandwich.*

- *Serve the sandwich by cutting it in half.*

STEAK SANDWICH, RATED

Information about diet:

There are four servings in this recipe. About 460 calories, 22 grams of fat, 36 grams of protein, and 30 grams of carbs are included in each sandwich.

10 minutes for preparation

15 minutes for cooking

<u>*Ingredients:*</u>

- *1 pound of thinly sliced cooked roast beef*
- *Four hoagies*
- *Four slices of provolone*
- *Sliced red onion, one*
- *1 sliced green bell pepper*
- *Pepper and salt as desired*
- *Olive oil, 2 tablespoons*

<u>*Makings:*</u>

- *Set your oven's temperature to 350 degrees Fahrenheit.*

- *Place the hoagie rolls on a baking pan after cutting them in half lengthwise.*

- *Apply olive oil to the rolls' inside.*

- *The rolls should be gently browned in the oven for 5-7 minutes.*

- *As the buns are toasting, soften and gently caramelize the red onion and green bell pepper in a skillet with a tablespoon of olive oil. To taste, add salt and pepper to the food.*

- *As soon as the veggies are cooked through, add the sliced roast meat to the pan and stir with them.*

- *Put a piece of provolone cheese on the bottom half of each bun after it has been toasted.*

- ***Spread the cheese with the roast beef mixture.***

- ***Add the second half of the bread to the sandwich's top.***

- ***Serving hot, please.***

A simple and fast dish that is great for lunch or supper is roast beef sandwiches. You can quickly prepare a nice sandwich using this recipe. Try experimenting with various cheeses, veggies, or sauces to give the dish your unique spin.

CHAPTER 6

RECIPES FOR SNACKS AND DESSERTS

BROUGHT APPLE CHIPS

Nutritional value:

This dish yields roughly 4 servings. Each serving has around 60 calories, 0 grams of fat, 16 grams of carbs, and 0 grams of protein. Depending on the size and variety of apples used, there may be variations in the precise nutritional content.

10 minutes for preparation
1 to 2 hours for cooking

<u>*Ingredients:*</u>

- ***Two big apples***
- ***A teaspoon of cinnamon***
- ***A spoonful of optional sugar***

<u>*Makings:*</u>

- ***Turn on the oven to 200 °F (93 °C).***

- ***Make thin slices of the apples using a mandolin or a knife.***
- ***If you'd like, you may either remove the skin or keep it on.***

- ***Combine the sugar (if using) and cinnamon in a small bowl.***

- *Apple slices should be arranged in a single layer on a baking sheet that has been lined with parchment paper.*
- *The cinnamon-sugar mixture is sprinkled over the apple slices.*

- *Bake the apple slices in the oven for one to two hours, or until crisp and golden. About halfway through the cooking process, turn the apple slices.*

- *Before serving, let the apple chips cool fully.*

Any time of day is a fantastic opportunity to enjoy baked apple chips as a snack. They are sweet, crunchy, and loaded with vitamins and fiber. Make a large batch so you can eat them all week long. They may be kept in an airtight jar for up to a week.

JELL-O WITH FRESH BERRIES AND NO SUGAR

Serving size: This dish yields around 4 servings.

This dish requires roughly 10 minutes of preparation time and two hours of refrigeration.

This dish requires around 10 minutes of preparation time.

Ingredients:

- *1 box of Jell-O sugar-free, any flavor*
- *2 cups of fresh berries, such as blueberries, strawberries, and raspberries*
- *4 cups of liquid*

Makings:

- *Remove any stems, leaves, or other debris before cleaning and preparing your fresh berries. Cut bigger berries into more manageable bits.*

- *Prepare the sugar-free Jell-O in a medium mixing bowl using 4 cups of water as directed on the container.*

- *Add the fresh berries to the bowl and gently swirl to blend when the Jell-O liquid has somewhat cooled.*

- *Fill individual serving plates or a larger serving dish with the mixture.*

- *The Jell-O should be chilled in the fridge for at least two hours, or until it is set.*

- *Dispense and savor.*

For individuals who are attempting to eat better or who are limiting their sugar consumption, this sugar-free Jell-O with fresh berries is a terrific dessert alternative. Fresh berries provide a healthy dose of antioxidants, and it's simple to prepare and low in calories. Enjoy it and give it a try for your next dessert!

UNSALTED NUTS AND SEEDS IN TRAIL MIX

Portion size

Approximately 6 cups of trail mix are produced by this recipe. A serving size of 1/4 cup is suggested, which has around 150 calories, 6 grams of protein, 11 grams of fat, 11 grams of carbs, and 2 grams of fiber.

Cooking Time: This meal has to be cooked for 8 to 10 minutes.

Preparation Time: Including the time it takes for the nuts to cool, this recipe's preparation takes around 10-15 minutes.

Nutritional Information

The unsalted nuts and seeds in this trail mix are a wonderful source of fiber, healthy fats, and protein. Additionally, it has no added sweeteners and minimal salt content.

Ingredients:

- *1 cup almonds without salt*
- *Unsalted cashews in a cup*
- *Unsalted peanuts in a cup*
- *Unseasoned pumpkin seeds, 1 cup*
- *Unsalted sunflower seeds in a cup*
- *1 cup of cranberries, dried*
- *100 g raisins*

Turn on the oven to 350 °F (175 °C).

On a baking sheet, spread the nuts in a single layer and roast for 8 to 10 minutes, or until gently toasted.
When the nuts are cooled, remove the baking sheet from the oven.

Combine the cooled nuts with the raisins, sunflower seeds, dried cranberries, and pumpkin seeds in a large mixing dish.

All of the ingredients should be well mixed.

In a cool, dry location, keep the trail mix in an airtight container.

SLICED BANANA AND ALMOND BUTTER IN A RICE CAKE

Size of serving: 1

5 minutes to prepare

0 minutes were spent cooking.

<u>*Ingredients:*</u>

- *One rice cake*
- *1/4 cup almond butter*
- *Sliced bananas, half*
- *Added extras include chia seeds, honey, and cinnamon.*

<u>*Makings:*</u>

- *Your rice cake should first be gently crisped up in a toaster or toaster oven.*

- *Apply the almond butter to the rice cake in an equal layers using a spoon or knife.*

- *Place the thinly sliced banana rounds on top of the almond butter.*

- *On top of the banana slices, you may optionally sprinkle chia seeds or cinnamon and pour in honey.*

- *While it's still warm and crispy, eat your rice cake with almond butter and sliced banana right away.*

Information about diet:

About 170 calories, 5 grams of protein, 26 grams of carbs, and 6 grams of fat are included in this dish. Fiber, potassium, and good fats from almond butter are all abundant in this food. In addition, the banana provides a boost of vitamins and minerals as well as natural sweetness.

LOW-SUGAR AND LOW-SODIUM BLUEBERRY OAT MUFFINS

12 muffins are served.

10 minutes for preparation

Time to cook: 20 minutes

Approximately 30 minutes.

Amounts of calories per serving:

- *146 calories*
- *Fat: 4.2g*

- *24.6g of carbohydrates*
- *2.5g of fiber*
- *4.2g of protein*
- *Salt: 66 mg*

Ingredients:

- *Old-fashioned oats, 1 1/2 cups*
- *All-purpose flour, 1 cup*
- *A half-cup of almond flour*
- *Quarter cup brown sugar*
- *Baking powder, two tablespoons*
- *A half-teaspoon of baking soda*
- *12 teaspoons each of salt and cinnamon*
- *2 eggs*
- *Unsweetened applesauce, half a cup*
- *Greek yogurt, plain, in 1/2 cup*
- *1/4 cup of almond milk without sugar*

> - *One cup of blueberries and one teaspoon of vanilla essence*

Makings:

- *Paper liners should be used to line a muffin pan while the oven is preheated to 375°F (190°C).*

- *Combine the oats, all-purpose flour, almond flour, brown sugar, baking soda, salt, and cinnamon in a large basin.*

- *Whisk the eggs, applesauce, Greek yogurt, almond milk, and vanilla extract into another dish.*

- *Just mix the dry components with the addition of the liquid ingredients.*

- *Fold the blueberries in slowly.*

- *Equally, distribute the batter among the 12 muffin tins.*

- *A toothpick placed in the center of the cake should come out clean after 20 minutes of baking.*

- *The muffins should cool in the pan for five minutes before being moved to a wire rack to finish cooling.*

Enjoy your blueberry oat muffins, which are low in sodium and sugar. For up to five days, keep any muffin leftovers in the refrigerator in an airtight container.

FROSTED GROVES

Nutritional information

There is no fat or cholesterol in one cup of frozen grapes, which has roughly 104 calories, 27 grams of carbs, and 1 gram of protein. Additionally, grapes are a significant source of potassium and vitamin C.

5 minutes for preparation

0 minutes were spent cooking.

Size of serving: 1 cup

Ingredients:

- *1 bag of grapes, fresh*

Makings:

- *The grapes should be carefully rinsed in cold water and dried with paper towels.*

- *The grapes' stems should be cut off.*

- *On a dish or baking sheet, arrange the grapes in a single layer.*

- *The grapes should be frozen entirely or for at least two hours after being placed in the freezer.*

- *When the grapes are frozen, move them to an airtight container or freezer bag and keep them there until you're ready to consume them.*

BURGUNDY CHICKPEAS

Cooking Time: The cooking will take 25 to 30 minutes in total.

The preparation for this meal takes just a few minutes.

Information on calories, protein, fiber, and carbs can be found in each serving of roasted chickpeas (1/4 cup), which has around 120 calories, 5 grams of protein, 5 grams of fiber, and 16 grams of carbohydrates.

Ingredients:

- *1 can (15 oz.) washed and drained chickpeas*
- *1 tablespoon of olive oil*
- *1/tsp. salt*
- *1 teaspoon cumin, ground*
- *1 teaspoon paprika*
- *12 teaspoons of garlic powder*

Makings:

- *For best results, line a baking sheet with parchment paper and preheat the oven to 400°F (200°C).*

- *With a paper towel, pat dry the chickpeas to get rid of any extra moisture.*

- *Combine the olive oil, salt, cumin, paprika, and garlic powder in a small bowl.*

- *When the chickpeas are completely covered in the spice mixture, add them to the bowl and toss them.*

- *On the baking sheet, distribute the chickpeas in a single layer.*

- *Bake the chickpeas for 20 to 25 minutes, or until they are crispy and golden brown.*

- *Before serving, take the chickpeas out of the oven and allow them cool for a while.*

- *Each serving of the four meals produced by this recipe contains around a quarter cup of roasted chickpeas.*

SODIUM-FREE POPCORN

This recipe yields enough low-sodium popcorn for four servings.

Cooking time: This meal has to be prepared in around 5 minutes.

Preparation: This dish requires around two minutes of preparation.

Ingredients:

- *Popcorn kernels, 1/2 cup*
- *Canola, coconut, or olive oil in the amount of two teaspoons*
- *Salt, 1/4 teaspoon*
- *Garlic powder, 1/4 teaspoon (optional)*

<u>*Makings:*</u>

- *Oil is added to a big pot that is already hot over medium-high heat.*

- *Popcorn kernels should be added to the saucepan after the oil is heated.*

- *Shake the pot and then cover it with a tight-fitting lid to spread the kernels evenly.*

- *As the popping slows down, let the kernels continue to pop while periodically shaking the pot.*

- *Turn off the heat and gently remove the cover from the saucepan.*

- *To equally distribute the salt and garlic powder, sprinkle it over the popcorn and toss.*

ALMOND MILK BERRY SMOOTHIE WITH LOW-POTASSIUM FRUITS

Serving Size: There are 2 servings in this dish.

Cooking Time: This dish doesn't need any cooking time.

Preparation Time: This dish requires around 10 minutes of preparation.

Approximately 220 calories, 4 grams of protein, 4 grams of fiber, and 22 grams of carbs are included in each serving of this smoothie.

Ingredients:

- *1 cup of strawberries, frozen*
- *1 cup of blueberries, frozen*
- *1 cup of almond milk without sugar*
- *Half a banana*

- *1 teaspoon of optional honey*

- *Ice cubes, if desired*

Makings:

- *Blenderize the frozen blueberries and strawberries.*

- *Add a banana that has been cut in half to the blender.*

- *Add 1 cup of almond milk without sugar.*

- *If preferred, add a spoonful of honey.*

- *The components should be well blended.*

- *Several ice cubes may be added to the smoothie if it is too thick. Blend again.*

- *Enjoy the smoothie by pouring it into two glasses.*

Smoothies with almond milk and low potassium content are a quick and delectable way to start the day. It makes for the ideal nutritious breakfast or snack since it is loaded with nutrients, fiber, and antioxidants. Additionally, you can easily personalize it by using your preferred low-potassium fruits and changing the sweetness to your preference. Try it out and take pleasure in a tasty and refreshing treat!

CHAPTER 7

AIR-FRYER RECIPE

FRIED SWEET POTATOES, BAKED

10 minutes for preparation

20 to 25 minutes for cooking

Dietary information (per serving):

- *150 calories*
- *Fat: 7g*
- *22g of carbohydrates*
- *3g of fiber*
- *2g protein*

Ingredients:

- *Two large sweet potatoes*
- *2/TBS of olive oil*
- *Garlic powder, 1 teaspoon*
- *1 teaspoon paprika*
- *Pepper and salt as desired*

Makings:

- *Set the oven's temperature to 425°F (218°C).*

- *The sweet potatoes should be peeled and then sliced into thin, even strips.*

- *Sweet potato strips should be mixed with olive oil, paprika, garlic powder, salt, and pepper in a large bowl.*

- *On a baking sheet, arrange the seasoned sweet potato fries in a single layer.*
- *Bake the fries for 20 to 25 minutes or until crispy and browned.*

- *Before serving, take the fries out of the oven and let them cool for a while.*

- *Depending on serving size, this recipe yields enough fries for two to three people.*

Throughout the day, baked sweet potato fries make a delicious side dish or snack. Try them and take advantage of all the advantages that sweet potatoes have to offer since they're simple to create, nutritious, and delectable.

SKEWERS OF GRILLED CHICKEN

Depending on the size of the chicken pieces and the number of veggies you use, this recipe yields around 6–8 skewers. Depending on the appetite of the individuals you are serving, the serving size will change.

The thickness of the chicken pieces and the heat of your grill will affect how long it takes to cook the grilled chicken skewers. It typically needs 10 to 15 minutes to cook completely, turning halfway through.

Preparation time: Grilled chicken skewers need just a brief amount of preparation. Making the ingredients and putting the skewers together will take around 20 to 30 minutes.

Nutritional information: With just 200 calories per serving, this meal is a lean and healthful choice. It has a high protein content and a low carbohydrate content. However, depending on the precise items you use, the nutritional information may change.

Ingredients:

- *1 pound of cut-up, skinless, boneless chicken breasts*
- *Cut one red bell pepper into 1-inch slices.*
- *1-inch-long slices of one yellow bell pepper*
- *Cut one red onion into 1-inch slices.*
- *Olive oil, two teaspoons*
- *Lemon juice, two teaspoons*
- *2 minced garlic cloves*
- *Oregano, dry, 1 teaspoon*
- *0.5 teaspoons of salt*
- *Black pepper, 1/4 teaspoon*
- *Wood skewers that have been submerged in water for at least 30 minutes*

Makings:

- *Heat the grill to medium-high.*

- *Olive oil, lemon juice, garlic, oregano, salt, and black pepper should all be combined in a small bowl.*

- *On skewers, alternately thread pieces of chicken, peppers, and onions.*

- *Apply the olive oil mixture on the skewers.*

- *The skewers should be placed on the grill and cooked for 10 to 15 minutes, turning them over halfway through.*

- *Remove from the grill, then warmly serve.*

Grilled chicken skewers are a quick and delicious dish that is ideal for any summer BBQ. They are a fantastic choice for individuals who wish to keep a balanced diet while enjoying a gourmet dinner since they are nutritious, low in fat, and rich in protein. Try this dish at your next barbecue to wow your guests with your grilling prowess!

GRILLED VEGGIES

Ingredients:

- *1 pound of your preferred veggies, such as bell peppers, onions, carrots, broccoli, cauliflower, sweet potatoes, etc.*
- *Olive oil, 2 tablespoons*
- *Pepper, and salt as desired*
- *Optional additions, such as dried herbs, paprika, onion powder, or garlic powder*

Makings:

Set the oven to 400 °F.

Your veggies should be washed and cut into bite-sized pieces.

Combine the chopped veggies, olive oil, salt, pepper, and any other spices in a large mixing dish. Toss the veggies until they are well covered.

On a baking sheet, arrange the veggies in a single layer.

The veggies should be roasted in the preheated oven for 20 to 30 minutes, stirring once or twice, or until they are soft and just beginning to brown.

For a filling and healthy supper, incorporate the roasted veggies into salads, wraps, or bowls. You can also serve them hot as a side dish.

Nutritional Information: Depending on the veggies used, this dish yields around 4 servings, each of which has 100–150 calories. Vegetables that have been roasted are a healthy complement to any meal since they are rich in fiber, vitamins, and minerals.

15 to 20 minutes for preparation
20–30 minutes for cooking
4 servings per item.

TACOS OF AIR-FRIED FISH

Four people may be fed with this dish.

Cooking time: This meal takes 20 to 25 minutes to prepare.

Preparation: This dish requires roughly 15 to 20 minutes of preparation.

Nutritional information: Each serving has around 300 calories, 30 grams of protein, 20 grams of carbs, 10 grams of fat, and 2 grams of fiber.

<u>Ingredients:</u>

- *White fish fillets weighing 1 lb., such as cod or tilapia*
- *All-purpose flour, half a cup*
- *Chili powder, 1 teaspoon*
- *1 teaspoon cumin*
- *12 teaspoon salt*
- *Black pepper, 1/4 teaspoon*
- *2 beaten eggs*
- *Panko breadcrumbs, 1 cup*
- *8 miniature tortillas*
- *1 diced avocado*
- *50% of a salsa.*
- *A half-cup of sour cream*
- *Wedges sliced from 1 lime*
- *Chopped fresh cilantro*

<u>*Makings:*</u>

Set your air fryer to 400°F for frying.

Combine the flour, cumin, salt, black pepper, and chili powder, and in a small bowl.

Fish fillets should be dipped in a flour mixture, beaten eggs, and then panko bread crumbs.

When the fish is cooked through and the breading is golden brown and crispy, place the breaded fish fillets in the air fryer basket and cook for 10 to 12 minutes, turning once halfway through.

Warm the tortillas in the microwave or on a griddle while the fish cooks.

Each tortilla should have a piece of fried fish on it before being topped with salsa, sliced avocado, and a dollop of sour cream. Each taco should be topped with a lime wedge and fresh cilantro.

Dispense and savor.

HUMMUS AND VEGGIE STICKS MADE AT HOME

Amounts of calories per serving:

- *260 calories*
- *19g total fat*
- *2.5g of saturated fat*
- *Salt: 210 mg*
- *17g of total carbs*
- *5g of dietary fiber*
- *2g of total sugars*
- *6g protein*

- *1 can of washed and drained chickpeas*
- *3 tablespoons of tahini*
- *2 minced garlic cloves*
- *Lemon juice, 1/4 cup*
- *Olive oil, 1/4 cup*
- *1 teaspoon cumin*
- *To taste, add salt and pepper.*
- *Sticks of cut carrots, celery, and bell peppers for dipping*

Makings:

- *Blend the chickpeas, tahini, garlic, lemon juice, olive oil, cumin, salt, and pepper in a food processor until they are smooth and creamy. A tablespoon of water at a time may be added to the hummus if it is too thick to get the ideal consistency.*

- *Serve the hummus in a dish with the vegetable sticks on the side for dipping.*

CHAPTER 8

SLOW COOKER RECIPES

CHICKEN AND VEGETABLE SOUP IN A SLOW COOKER

Six servings per recipe

6 to 8 hours for cooking

15 minutes for preparation

<u>*Information about diet:*</u>

- *213 calories*
- *Fat total: 3.7g*
- *0.8g of saturated fat*
- *47 mg. cholesterol*
- *Salt: 736 mg*
- *21.7g of carbohydrates overall*
- *5.2g of dietary fiber*
- *7.5g of sugars*
- *24.8g of protein*

<u>*Ingredients:*</u>

- *One pound of cut-up, skinless, boneless chicken breasts*

* *1 medium sweet potato, peeled and chopped 1 big onion, chopped 3 cloves of garlic, minced 2 medium carrots, chopped 2 stalks of celery, chopped 1 can of diced tomatoes, with juices*
* *1 teaspoon dried thyme in 4 cups of chicken broth*
* *1 teaspoon dried rosemary*
* *Bay leaf, one*
* *To taste, add salt and pepper.*
* *Baby spinach leaves in 2 cups*

Makings:

* *Chicken, onion, garlic, carrots, celery, sweet potatoes, diced tomatoes, chicken broth, thyme, rosemary, bay leaf, salt, and pepper should all be combined in a slow cooker.*

* *Cook on low for 6 to 8 hours, or until the chicken is cooked through and the veggies are soft.*

- *Remove and discard the bay leaf.*

- *Baby spinach leaves should be added to the slow cooker and stirred for a couple of minutes until wilted.*

- *Serving hot, please.*

TURKEY CHILLI IN SLOW COOKER

Depending on the size of your slow cooker, this recipe yields around 6 to 8 servings. This dish takes around 15-20 minutes to prepare, and it takes 6-8 hours on low or 3-4 hours on high to cook.

Nutrition value:

- *258 calories*

- *5g total fat*

- *1g of saturated fat*

- *42 mg cholesterol*

- *554 milligrams of sodium*

- *28g of total carbohydrates*

- *9g of dietary fiber*

- *7g of total sugars*

- *25g of protein*

Ingredients:

- *1 pound of turkey, ground*

- *One sliced onion*

- *3 minced garlic cloves*

- *1 sliced bell pepper, 1 can of washed and drained kidney beans*

- *1 tomato-diced can*

- *10 grams of chili powder*

- *1 teaspoon of cumin, ground*

- *Paprika, half a teaspoon*

- *To taste, add salt and pepper.*

- *Optional garnishes: sour cream, chopped cilantro, and grated cheese*

<u>*Makings:*</u>

- *The ground turkey is added to a pan that is already hot over medium-high heat. Cook until browned, using a wooden spoon to break up any big bits.*

- *To the slow cooker, add the cooked turkey, onion, garlic, bell pepper, kidney beans, chopped tomatoes, cumin, paprika, chili powder, salt, and pepper.*

- *Everything should be well mixed together.*

- *Cook the slow cooker with the lid on for 6 to 8 hours on low heat or 3 to 4 hours on high heat.*

- *Cooked chili should be tasted and any necessary seasoning adjustments made.*

- *If wanted, top with your preferred toppings and serve hot.*

PORK TENDERLOIN IN SLOW COOKER WITH APPLES AND SWEET POTATOES

This recipe makes enough for four people to eat it.

Cooking Time: In a slow cooker, this recipe has to be cooked for around 4-6 hours on low heat.

Preparation Time: This dish requires around 15 minutes of preparation time.

<u>*Nutritional Information:*</u> There are around 400 calories, 35 grams of protein, 40 grams of carbs, and 10 grams of fat in each serving of this pork tenderloin with apples and sweet potatoes from the slow cooker.

<u>*Ingredients:*</u>

- ***2 1-pound each pork tenderloins***
- ***2 peeled and sliced slices of sweet potatoes***
- ***Peeled and cut into slices, two apples***
- ***One sliced onion***
- ***Apple cider vinegar, 1/4 cup***
- ***Honey, 1/4 cup***
- ***1/fourth cup of Dijon mustard***
- ***1 teaspoon of cinnamon powder***
- ***1/8 teaspoon of ginger root powder***

- *To taste, add salt and pepper.*

<u>*Makings:*</u>

- *Combine the apple cider vinegar, honey, Dijon mustard, cinnamon, ginger, salt, and pepper in a small bowl.*

- *In the slow cooker, put the pork tenderloins. Make careful to cover all sides of the pork, and pour the mixture over it.*

- *Place the pork in the center of the slow cooker and then add the cut sweet potatoes, apples, and onions.*

- *Cook the pork on low heat for 4-6 hours, or until it is soft and cooked through, with the cover on the slow cooker.*

- *Put the cooked pork on a chopping board after removing it from the slow cooker. Before cutting it into pieces, let it sit for a while.*

- *Serve the pork with the apples and sweet potatoes while dousing everything with sauce.*

BEEF STEW IN THE SLOW COOKER WITH ROOT VEGETABLES

It takes 15 minutes to prepare and 8 hours to cook this meal, which feeds 6 people. The nutritional facts per serving are as follows:

- *398 calories*
- *Fat: 12g*
- *3g of saturated fat*
- *97mg of cholesterol*

* *Salt: 952 mg*

* *28g of carbohydrates*

* *5g of fiber*

* *Sucrose: 5g*

* *42g of protein*

Ingredients:

* *2 pounds of cubed, 1-inch-wide beef stew meat*

* *2 tablespoons of regular flour*

* *1 salt shaker*

* *Black pepper, half a teaspoon*

* *Olive oil, two teaspoons*

* *1 tablespoon tomato paste in 2 cups of beef broth*

* *A serving of Worcestershire sauce*

* *1 diced onion, 4 minced garlic cloves*

* *4 sliced and peeled carrots*

* *2 peeled and sliced parsnips*

- *2 chopped and peeled potatoes*
- *Two cups of beef stock*
- *1 teaspoon dried thyme, 2 bay leaves*

Makings:

- *Combine the flour, salt, and black pepper in a bowl. Incorporate the meat cubes and stir to coat.*

- *In a large skillet over medium-high heat, warm the olive oil.*

- *Add the meat and cook it until it is well-browned all over.*

- *Put the steak in the slow cooker. Onions, garlic, carrots, parsnips, potatoes, tomato paste, Worcestershire sauce, beef broth, bay leaves, and thyme should all be added.*

- *Cook the meat and veggies in the slow cooker with the lid on for 8 hours on low or 4 hours on high, depending on your preference.*

- *Serve hot after removing the bay leaves.*

A rich and soothing dish like Slow Cooker Beef Stew with Root Vegetables is ideal for a relaxing evening at home. A tasty and filling stew is produced as a consequence of the flavors coming together slowly while cooking.

LENTIL SOUP IN SLOW COOKER WITH SPINACH AND CARROTS

Servings: six

8 hours for cooking

15 minutes for preparation

<u>*Dietary information (per serving):*</u>

- **215 calories**
- **Fat: 1g**
- **42g of carbohydrates**
- **18g of fiber**
- **15g of protein**

<u>*Ingredients:*</u>

- **One sliced onion**
- **2 diced carrots, 2 chopped celery stalks, and 3 minced garlic cloves**
- **1 teaspoon each of ground cumin and coriander**
- **One tablespoon of dried thyme**
- **Bay leaf, one**
- **1 cup of washed and drained dry brown lentils**
- **4 cups of veggie broth**

- *Chopped tomatoes in a single 14.5-ounce can*

- *1 salt shaker*

- *Black pepper, 1/4 teaspoon*

- *2 cups freshly cleaned and cut spinach leaves*

- *One teaspoon of lemon juice*

Makings:

- *Combine the lentils, vegetable broth, diced tomatoes, salt, and black pepper in a slow cooker along with the onion, carrots, celery, garlic, cumin, coriander, thyme, and bay leaf.*

- *Combine all ingredients by stirring.*

- *Cook covered for 8 hours on low or 4 hours on high.*

- *Add the chopped spinach and lemon juice to the slow cooker, then stir to incorporate about 30 minutes before the soup is ready.*

- *For an extra 30 minutes, cook with a cover.*

- *Before serving, throw away the bay leaf.*

- *Serving hot, please.*

CHAPTER 9

INSTANT-POT RECIPES

CHICKEN NOODLE SOUP IN A DISH

A tasty and nourishing dinner that can be prepared quickly and effortlessly in a pressure cooker is instant pot chicken noodle soup. It takes 15 minutes to prepare and 25 minutes to cook this meal, which serves 6.

Per-serving nutritional information:

- *315 calories*
- *Fat: 8g*
- *28g of protein*

- *30g of carbohydrates*

- *3g of fiber*

- *4g sugar*

- *1020 milligrams of sodium*

Ingredients:

- *Olive oil, 1 tbsp.*

- *1 diced onion, 3 minced garlic cloves*

- *Chop three carrots, three celery stalks, and one pound of skinless, boneless chicken breasts.*

- *8 cups of chicken stock*

- *Two cups of egg noodles*

- *One tablespoon of dried thyme*

- *To taste, add salt and pepper.*

- *Fresh parsley, chopped, as a garnish (optional)*

Makings:

- *Select the "sauté" option on the Instant Pot and turn it on. Olive oil is added, and it is heated for a minute. Once the onion is transparent, add the garlic and continue cooking for a few minutes.*

- *Cook the carrots and celery in the saucepan for a further two to three minutes.*

- *Add the chicken breasts, egg noodles, dried thyme, chicken broth, salt, and pepper to the saucepan.*

- *Close the cover and program the Instant Pot to cook for 15 minutes at high pressure.*

- *Use the quick-release technique to relieve the pressure when the cooking period has ended.*

- ***Remove the chicken breasts by lifting the cover. The chicken should be shredded with two forks before being added back to the saucepan.***

The soup should be stirred and given some time to thicken. After that, serve in dishes and, if you like, top with freshly cut parsley.

A warm and nutritious dinner like Instant Pot Chicken Noodle Soup is ideal for a chilly day or when you're feeling under the weather. It's simple to prepare and adaptable to your preferences by using more veggies or seasonings.

POT RED LENTIL CHILLI, IMMEDIATE

The recipe makes plenty for 4-6 people.

10 minutes for preparation

10 minutes for cooking

Approximately 20 minutes.

<u>*Per-serving nutritional information (based on 6 servings):*</u>

- **240 calories**
- **4g total fat**
- **0.5g of saturated fat**
- **0 mg of cholesterol**
- **Salt: 471 mg**
- **38g of total carbohydrates**
- **13g of dietary fiber**
- **5g of total sugars**
- **14g of protein**

<u>*Ingredients:*</u>

- **Olive oil, 1 tbsp.**
- **Diced one medium onion**
- **3 minced garlic cloves**

- *10 grams of chili powder*

- *1 teaspoon of cumin, ground*

- *A half-teaspoon of smoked paprika*

- *Cayenne pepper, 1/4 teaspoon (optional)*

- *1 cup of washed and drained red lentils*

- *15 ounces of chopped tomatoes in a can, untrained*

- *Two cups of vegetable stock*

- *1 can (15 ounces) of washed and drained kidney beans*

- *To taste, add salt and pepper.*

- *Fresh cilantro, chopped, as a garnish (optional)*

<u>Makings:</u>

- *Heat the olive oil in your Instant Pot by pressing the sauté button. Stirring periodically, add the onion and garlic, and cook until tender.*

- *Cook for 1 minute while continually whisking in the chili powder, cumin, smoked paprika, and cayenne pepper (if using).*

- *Stir in the vegetable broth, diced tomatoes, and red lentils after adding them.*

- *Set the valve to the sealing position and lock the lid in place. 10 minutes of high-pressure cooking.*

- *After the cooking process is finished, let the pressure naturally relax for 10 minutes before manually releasing any leftover pressure.*

- *Add the kidney beans after seasoning to taste with salt and pepper. If desired, add cilantro as a garnish.*

POT BALSAMIC CHICKEN IN A MINUTE

This dish takes around 10 minutes to prepare and 25 minutes to cook, and it feeds 4 people. About 230 calories, 3 grams of fat, 17 grams of carbs, and 32 grams of protein are included in each serving.

Ingredients:

- *1 lb. of skinless, boneless chicken breasts*
- *Balsamic vinegar, half a cup*
- *1/fourth cup of chicken broth*
- *Honey, two tablespoons*
- *2 minced garlic cloves*
- *One tablespoon of dried basil*
- *To taste, add salt and pepper.*
- *Corn flour, one tablespoon*
- *1 teaspoon of water*

- *Add-on garnish: fresh parsley or green onions, chopped*

<u>*Makings:*</u>

- *Starting in the Instant Pot, combine the balsamic vinegar, chicken broth, honey, garlic, dried basil, salt, and pepper. To blend, stir.*

- *Make sure the chicken breasts are well soaked in the liquid before adding them to the saucepan.*

- *Put the Instant Pot's cover on and program it to cook for 10 minutes at high pressure.*

- *After the allotted cooking time has passed, give the pressure a five-minute natural release before using the rapid release to relieve any leftover pressure.*

- *Place the chicken on a chopping board after removing it from the Instant Pot. To shred the chicken into tiny pieces, use two forks.*

- *In the meanwhile, create a slurry by mixing corn flour and water in a small bowl.*
- *Stir the corn flour slurry into the Instant Pot while it is on the sauté setting. Cook the sauce, stirring often, for 2 to 3 minutes, or until it thickens.*

- *Stir to mix the shredded chicken in the thickened sauce before adding it back to the stove.*

- *If preferred, top the hot Instant Pot Balsamic Chicken with chopped fresh parsley or green onions.*

BEEF STEW INSTANT POT

<u>*Ingredients:*</u>

- *2 minced garlic cloves*
- *One tablespoon of dried thyme*
- *1 paprika teaspoon*
- *1 salt shaker*
- *Black pepper, half a teaspoon*
- *Corn flour, two teaspoons*
- *Water in 2 tablespoons*

<u>*Makings:*</u>

- *Place the steak in the Instant Pot's sauté setting. The meat should be cooked for a few minutes until browned on both sides. The meat should be taken out of the Instant Pot and left aside.*

- *In the Instant Pot, combine the onion, carrots, potatoes, beef broth, tomato paste, garlic, thyme, paprika, salt, and pepper. To blend, stir.*

- *Stirring the other ingredients together, add the meat back to the Instant Pot.*

- *Set the valve to "sealing" and close the Instant Pot lid. 35 minutes of high-pressure cooking.*

- *Allow the pressure to naturally relax for 10 minutes after the cooking process is finished, then quickly remove any leftover pressure.*

- *Corn flour and water should be well whipped together in a small bowl. To thicken the stew in the Instant Pot, stir in the corn flour mixture.*

- *If preferred, top the hot beef stew with fresh parsley before serving.*

Nutritional information: Each serving of this Instant Pot beef stew has around 400 calories, 30 grams of protein, 25 grams of carbs, and 20 grams of fat. Iron, vitamin A, and potassium are all found in abundance in the stew.

Enjoy your tasty and simple beef stew made in the Instant Pot.

TURKEY MEATBALLS IN A MINUTE

8 minutes of high-pressure cooking.

Allow the Instant Pot to naturally reduce pressure for five minutes after the cooking cycle is finished, then quickly release any leftover pressure.

Serve the meatballs hot with more Parmesan cheese and parsley, if wanted, after carefully removing the cover.

Food and nutrition facts (per serving):

- *191 calories*
- *Fat: 9g*
- *2g of saturated fat*
- *81 milligrams of cholesterol.*
- *554 milligrams of sodium*
- *8g of carbohydrates*
- *1g of fiber*
- *3g of sugar*
- *19g of protein*

Ingredients:

- *1 pound of turkey meat*
- *A half-cup of breadcrumbs*

- *Parmesan cheese, grated, in 1/4 cup; fresh parsley, minced, in 1/4 cup*
- *One egg and a teaspoon of garlic powder*
- *1/4 teaspoon black pepper and 1/2 teaspoon salt*
- *One water cup*
- *1 cup of sauce for pasta*

Makings:

- *Combine the ground turkey, breadcrumbs, Parmesan cheese, parsley that has been chopped, egg, garlic powder, salt, and pepper in a large mixing basin. Mix thoroughly.*

- *Form the mixture into little meatballs using a tablespoon or a small cookie scoop.*

- *After adding the meatballs and making sure they are spread equally, pour the water into the Instant Pot.*

- *Make sure to completely cover all of the meatballs with the marinara sauce as you pour it over them.*

- *Set the valve to the sealing position and close the Instant Pot lid.*

CHAPTER 10

SOUP AND STEW

SOUP WITH CHICKEN AND VEGETABLES

This dish yields enough food for four persons.

Cooking Time: The cooking will take 40 to 45 minutes in total.

Preparation Time: It takes around 15 to 20 minutes to prepare.

Each serving of this soup has around 250–300 calories, 25–30 grams of protein, 20–25 grams of carbs, and 8–10 grams of fat.

Ingredients:

- *1 lb. of skinless, boneless chicken breasts*
- *Olive oil, two teaspoons*
- *One sliced onion*
- *2 minced garlic cloves*

- *2 cups of chopped mixed veggies, such as green beans, carrots, and celery*

- *6 cups of chicken stock*

- *Bay leaf, one*

- *To taste, add salt and pepper.*

- *Chopped fresh parsley is optional.*

Makings:

- *Start by bringing the olive oil to medium-high heat in a big saucepan or Dutch oven.*

- *Add the onion and garlic, and cook for approximately 5 minutes, or until they are tender.*

- *Sauté for a further five minutes after adding the chopped veggies.*

- *Bring the mixture to a boil before adding the chicken broth and bay leaf.*

- *Add the chicken breasts to the saucepan and turn the heat down.*

- *The chicken should be cooked through after 15 to 20 minutes of cooking under cover.*

- *Use two forks to shred the chicken after removing it from the saucepan.*

- *Re-add the chicken that has been shredded into the saucepan, then season with salt & pepper to taste.*

- *To let the flavors combine, simmer the soup for an extra 10-15 minutes.*

- *If preferred, garnish the hot soup with fresh parsley after removing the bay leaf.*

Chicken and vegetable soup is a tasty, wholesome, and simple dish. You can prepare a filling and healthy supper that will keep you satisfied and content for hours with only a few basic items and some time.

LEMON SOUP

- *Size of serving: 1 1/2 cups*
- *30 minutes for cooking*
- *10 minutes for preparation*

- *Amounts of calories per serving:*
- *260 calories*
- *7g of total fat*
- *1g of saturated fat*
- *0 mg of cholesterol*
- *Salt: 824 mg*

- *37g of total carbs*

- *15g of dietary fiber*

- *6g sugars*

- *14g of protein*

Ingredients:

- *1 cup of washed and drained dry lentils*
- *2 minced garlic cloves and 1 chopped onion*
- *Two sliced carrots and two chopped celery stalks*
- *4 cups of veggie stock*
- *One tomato chopped in a can*
- *1 teaspoon of cumin powder*
- *Oregano, dry, 1 teaspoon*
- *Olive oil and two teaspoons of salt and pepper, to taste*

Makings:

- *Over medium heat, warm the olive oil in a big saucepan. When the onion is transparent, add the garlic and onion.*

- *Cook the carrots and celery for a further five minutes after adding them.*

- *Cumin, oregano, chopped tomatoes, lentils, and vegetable broth should all be added. Once it starts to boil, turn the heat down, cover, and simmer for approximately 30 minutes, or until the lentils are cooked.*

- *To taste, add salt and pepper to the food.*

- *Use an immersion blender to puree the soup to your preferred consistency if you like a smoother texture.*

- *Serving hot, please.*

A full and healthy meal, lentil soup may be eaten as a main course or a side dish. You may easily alter it by using your preferred veggies or seasonings. Additionally, it's a fantastic way to use up refrigerator leftover veggies. Try it and take advantage of lentils' beneficial health properties!

BUFFALO STEW

The beef stew in this recipe serves six people.

Preparation Time: This dish requires around 20 minutes of preparation time.

Cooking Time: This dish takes between 2.5 and 3 hours to prepare.

Nutritional Information: This beef stew has around 350 calories per serving, 24 grams of protein, and 13 grams of fat.

Ingredients:

- ***1-inch chunks of beef chuck, weighing 2 pounds.***
- ***Two teaspoons of regular flour***
- ***Olive oil, 2 tablespoons***
- ***1 big, chopped onion***
- ***3 minced garlic cloves***
- ***Two cups of beef stock***
- ***Water, 1 cup***
- ***2 teaspoons of dried thyme and 1 bay leaf***
- ***4 sliced carrots***
- ***3 peeled and sliced potatoes***
- ***To taste, add salt and pepper.***
- ***For decoration, chop some parsley.***

<u>*Makings:*</u>

- *The beef cubes should first be floured. As the stew cooks, this will assist in making it thicker.*

- *Over medium-high heat, warm the olive oil in a big saucepan or Dutch oven. Add the steak, then sear it well.*

- *The meat should be taken out of the saucepan and kept aside.*

- *When the onions are translucent, add the onion and garlic to the saucepan and sauté for a few minutes.*

- *Add the water, bay leaf, thyme, beef broth, and meat back to the saucepan. To blend, stir.*

- *As soon as the mixture comes to a boil, turn the heat down to low and cover the pan. Give the stew 1.5 to 2 hours to cook.*

- *Stir together the potatoes and carrots after adding them to the saucepan. Cover the pan and simmer for another hour, or until the meat is well cooked and the veggies are soft.*

- *Add salt and pepper to taste while preparing the stew. Get rid of the bay leaf.*

- *Serve the beef stew hot with chopped parsley as a garnish.*

MEAT SOUP

Nutrition information:

- *170 calories*
- *Fat: 10g*
- *18g of carbohydrates*
- *4g. protein*
- *Salt: 1280 mg*
- *4g of fiber*

Ingredients:

- *Olive oil, 1 tbsp.*
- *1 diced onion, 2 minced garlic cloves*
- *Two 28-ounce cans of crushed tomatoes*
- *2 cups chicken or veggie broth 1 tsp. dried basil*
- *Oregano, dry, 1 teaspoon*
- *1 salt shaker*
- *Black pepper, 1/4 teaspoon*
- *50 ml of thick cream*

<u>*Makings:*</u>

- *Olive oil should be heated in a large saucepan over medium heat. Cook the onion and garlic for approximately 5 minutes, or until tender.*

- *Crushed tomatoes, chicken or vegetable broth, dried basil, dried oregano, salt, and black pepper should all be added. Bring to a boil, then turn down the heat. For 20 to 25 minutes, let simmer.*

- *To purée the soup until it is smooth, either use an immersion blender or transfer it to a blender.*

- *Add the heavy cream, then heat through for a further 5 minutes.*

- *Serving hot, please.*

SOUP WITH GINGER AND CARROT

This dish yields around 4-6 servings.

15 minutes or so for preparation.

The time needed to cook: around 25 minutes.

Nutritional information: This soup has around 160 calories per serving, 4 grams of protein, 16 grams of carbs, 10 grams of fat, 4 grams of fiber, and 7 grams of sugar.

Ingredients:

- *Olive oil, 1 tbsp.*
- *One sliced onion*
- *1 teaspoon grated ginger*
- *1 pound of sliced carrots and 4 cups of vegetable broth*

- *Coconut milk, 1 cup*

- *To taste, add salt and pepper.*

Makings:

- *Over medium heat, warm the olive oil in a big saucepan. Once the onion is tender and transparent, add the ginger as well.*

- *Vegetable broth and chopped carrots should be added to the saucepan. After bringing the mixture to a boil, lower the heat to a simmer. The carrots should be soft after 20 to 25 minutes of cooking under cover.*

- *Until the soup is creamy, mix it using an immersion blender.*

- *You may puree the soup in batches with a conventional blender if you don't have an immersion blender.*

- *Add the coconut milk after seasoning to taste with salt and pepper.*

- *Enjoy the soup while it's still hot.*

SOUP MINESTRONE

6–8 servings per recipe

30-45 minutes for cooking

15-20 minutes for preparation

Per-serving nutritional information (based on 6 servings):

- *210 calories*

- *Fat: 3g*

- *37g of carbohydrates*
- *10g of protein*
- *9g of fiber*

Ingredients:

- *Olive oil, 1 tbsp.*
- *1 diced onion*
- *3 minced garlic cloves, 2 chopped carrots, 2 diced celery stalks, and 1 sliced zucchini*
- *14 oz. can of chopped tomatoes*
- *4 cups of veggie stock*
- *1 can of washed and drained white beans*
- *One cup of little pasta*
- *2 cups of spinach or kale, chopped*
- *Pepper and salt as desired*
- *Parmesan cheese, if desired*

Makings:

- *Olive oil should be heated in a large saucepan over medium heat. Add the onion and garlic, then cook until they are tender.*

- *Add the zucchini, celery, and carrots and sauté for an additional 5 minutes, or until the veggies are just beginning to soften.*

- *White beans, vegetable broth, and diced tomatoes should all be added to the saucepan. After bringing it to a simmer, cook for 10 to 15 minutes.*

- *When the pasta is ready, add it and boil for a little longer.*

- *When the kale or spinach has wilted, add it and stir.*

- *To taste, add salt and pepper to the food.*

- *If preferred, top the heated dish with a little Parmesan cheese.*

Any veggies you have on hand may be used to make the adaptable meal known as minestrone. It's a wonderful way to get your recommended serving of veggies each day and is ideal for a warm lunch on a cold day.

PIZZA STEW

Amounts of calories per serving:

- *225 calories*
- *Fat: 7g*
- *27g of protein*
- *14g of carbohydrates*
- *3g of fiber*

- *Sucrose: 6g*
- *Salt: 804 mg*

Ingredients:

- *Cod, halibut, or any firm white fish weighing 1 pound*
- *One tomato chopped in a can*
- *One sliced onion*
- *3 minced garlic cloves*
- *1 chopped red bell pepper*
- *Olive oil, 1 tbsp.*
- *Paprika, 1 teaspoon*
- *Cumin, 1 teaspoon*
- *A pinch of salt*
- *Black pepper, half a teaspoon*
- *2 cups of fish or vegetable stock*
- *Chopped one-fourth cup of fresh parsley*

- *In a big saucepan, warm up the olive oil over medium heat.*

- *Cook the red bell pepper, onion, and garlic for 5 minutes, or until the vegetables are tender.*

- *Stir in the paprika, cumin, salt, and black pepper after adding them to the saucepan.*

- *Bring to a boil after adding the chopped tomatoes and vegetable or fish stock.*

- *Add the fish to the saucepan after lowering the heat. Simmer the fish for 10 to 15 minutes, or until it is fully cooked and flaky.*

- *Stir in the parsley after adding it to the saucepan.*

- *Pour the stew into bowls and serve it hot with rice or crusty bread.*

Fish stew is a tasty, nutritious, and simple dish to make. You may make a great supper that will wow your family and friends with only a few basic components.

CROSS PEA SOUP

10 minutes for preparation
1 hour for cooking
1 hour and 10 minutes in total

Ingredients:

- *Dried split peas, two cups*

- *8 cups of liquid*

- *1 teaspoon dried thyme, 2 medium onions, diced, 2 garlic cloves, minced, 2 celery stalks, chopped, and 2 carrots, chopped.*
- *Bay leaf, one*
- *To taste, add salt and pepper.*
- *Olive oil, two teaspoons*

Info about nutrition:

- *Size of serving: 1 cup*
- *187 calories*
- *Fat: 3g*
- *32g of carbohydrates*
- *13g of fiber*
- *11g of protein*

Makings:

- *The split peas should be rinsed before being added to a big saucepan with 8 cups of water.*

- *After bringing it to a boil, lower the heat, and let the mixture simmer for 30 minutes.*

- *Olive oil should be heated in a separate pan over medium heat.*

- *Add the carrots, celery, onions, and garlic. Cook the veggies for 10 to 15 minutes, or until they are tender.*

- *To the split peas and veggies in the saucepan, add the cooked vegetables.*

- *Add the salt, pepper, bay leaf, and thyme. Continue simmering for a further 30 minutes, or until the split peas are cooked through.*

- *After removing the bay leaf, smooth down the soup using an immersion blender.*

- *Alternatively, you may use a standard blender, but be sure to wait until the soup has cooled to prevent burning yourself.*

- *Serve hot with crackers or crusty toast.*

SOUP WITH SWEET POTATO AND KALE

Ingredients:

- *2 big, peeled, and chopped sweet potatoes*
- *1 bunch of chopped and cleaned kale*
- *1 diced onion, 2 minced garlic cloves*
- *4 cups of veggie stock*
- *Coconut milk, 1 cup*

Makings:

- *Over medium heat, warm the olive oil in a big saucepan.*

- *When the onions are transparent, add the minced garlic and onions and sauté for a further two to three minutes.*

- *Stir the onions and garlic into the stew before adding the sweet potatoes.*

- *Bring the mixture to a boil after adding the veggie broth.*

- *When the sweet potatoes are ready, turn the heat down to low and let the soup simmer for approximately 20 minutes.*

- *When the kale is wilted, add the chopped kale to the saucepan and simmer for an additional 5-7 minutes.*

- *After removing the soup from the heat source, wait a few minutes before serving. The soup should then be blended with a conventional blender or an immersion blender until it is creamy and smooth.*

- *Refill the pot with the soup, then whisk in the coconut milk. Add salt and pepper to taste and continue to reheat the soup over low heat.*

- *Along with a piece of crusty bread, serve the soup hot.*

- *With preparation and cooking time, this meal takes around 40 minutes to prepare and serves 4-6 people.*

(Based on 4 servings) Nutritional Information per Serving:

- *290 calories*
- *Fat: 15g*
- *35g of carbohydrates*
- *7g of fiber*
- *5g protein*

A tasty and nutritious recipe that is ideal for lunch or supper is sweet potato and kale soup. This soup is a fantastic choice for anyone with dietary limitations since it is vegan, gluten-free, and dairy-free.

SOUP WITH WHITE BEANS AND VEGETABLES

This recipe makes enough for four people to eat it.

Cooking time: This meal takes around 45 minutes to prepare.

Preparation: This dish requires roughly 15 minutes of preparation.

About 270 calories, 15 grams of protein, 50 grams of carbs, 7 grams of fiber, and 2 grams of fat are included in each serving of this soup.

Ingredients:

- *Olive oil, 1 tbsp.*

- *1 chopped onion, 2 minced garlic cloves, 3 peeled and diced carrots, 2 chopped celery stalks, 1 chopped red bell pepper, 4 cups vegetable broth, and 2 cans of rinsed and drained white beans*
- *One tablespoon of dried thyme*
- *Oregano, dry, 1 teaspoon*
- *Pepper and salt as desired*

<u>*Makings:*</u>

- *Olive oil should be heated in a large saucepan over medium heat.*

- *When the onion is transparent, add the garlic and onion and sauté for approximately 5 minutes.*

- *For a further 5 minutes, add the carrots, celery, and red bell pepper to the saucepan and sauté.*

- *Stir together the white beans, vegetable broth, thyme, and oregano in the saucepan.*

- *The soup should be brought to a boil, then simmered for approximately 30 minutes, or until the veggies are fork-tender.*

- *Add salt and pepper to taste while preparing the soup.*

- *Serving hot, please.*

CHAPTER 11

HEALTHY EATING ADVICE FOR PEOPLE WITH KIDNEY DISEASE

Having a good diet is important for everyone, but having kidney illness makes it even more important. Because their kidneys are no longer as effective at removing waste and extra fluids, people with renal disease need to be cautious about what they eat and drink. This may cause the body to accumulate hazardous amounts of poisons and other chemicals.

Working closely with your individualized dietary plan that addresses your unique requirements is crucial if you have renal disease. A kidney-healthy diet is often one that is high in vitamins, minerals, and fiber, but low in salt, phosphorus, and protein.

Here are some recommendations for eating well if you have renal disease:

✓ **_Aim to limit your salt consumption._**

Blood pressure increases caused by sodium might damage your kidneys. As a result, it's critical to keep your daily salt consumption to a maximum of 2,300 milligrams.

Avoiding processed meals, canned items, and other high-sodium foods can help you accomplish this. Instead, choose healthy grains, lean meats, fresh or frozen fruits and vegetables, and low-sodium spices.

✓ **_Your Phosphorous Intake Is Under Control_**

Your kidneys can't get rid of extra phosphorus from your body when they're not working correctly. Bone deterioration and other health issues may result from eating too much phosphorus.

Avoid high-phosphorus foods like dairy, nuts, and seeds if you want to keep your phosphorus consumption under control. Additionally, since they often include phosphoric acid, processed meals, and fizzy drinks should be avoided.

✓ *Try to consume less proteins.*

While necessary for tissue growth and repair, protein may be detrimental to your kidneys. Protein waste products may accumulate in your body and harm your kidneys if your kidneys are unable to clear them.

As a result, it's crucial to keep your daily protein consumption at 0.8 grams per kilogram of body weight. This may be accomplished by minimizing your consumption of red meat and opting for lean foods like chicken, fish, and tofu.

✓ **_Pick fruits and vegetables that are gentle on the kidneys._**

A healthy diet should include fruits and vegetables, but some of them may be heavy in potassium or phosphorus, which might damage your kidneys. Fruits and vegetables that are good for the kidneys include apples, blueberries, cherries, cranberries, red grapes, cabbage, and

Peppers, cauliflower, eggplant, and zucchini. The fruits and vegetables that are safe for you to consume should be discussed with your dietician.

✓ **_Take in a lot of water._**

Your body may retain extra fluids if you have a renal illness. It's crucial to consume enough water to assist flush out these fluids. Aim for eight glasses of water or more each day, unless your doctor has advised you to consume less water.

✓ *Observe portion sizes.*

Any meal in excess may be dangerous, but renal disease sufferers are more at risk. Because of this, it's crucial to keep an eye on your portion sizes and eat smaller, more frequent meals throughout the day. To make sure you're consuming the appropriate quantity of food, you may also use a scale or measuring cups.

✓ *Make your food*

You have greater control over what goes into your diet when you prepare your meals. You may choose natural, nutritious ingredients and control how much salt, phosphorus, and protein you consume. Additionally, preparing your food may be a creative and entertaining way to try different flavors and cultures.

✓ *Read the food labels.*

Be important to carefully read food labels when you go grocery shopping. To prevent consuming too much salt, phosphorus, or protein, look for goods that are low in these nutrients.